Alexander John Wedderbrun

**A Compilation of the Pharmacy and Drug Laws**

Of the Several States and Territories

Alexander John Wedderbrun

**A Compilation of the Pharmacy and Drug Laws**
*Of the Several States and Territories*

ISBN/EAN: 9783337232641

Printed in Europe, USA, Canada, Australia, Japan

Cover: Foto ©Suzi / pixelio.de

More available books at **www.hansebooks.com**

Bulletin No. 42

# U. S. DEPARTMENT OF AGRICULTURE
## DIVISION OF CHEMISTRY

# A COMPILATION

## OF THE

# PHARMACY AND DRUG LAWS

## OF THE

## SEVERAL STATES AND TERRITORIES

BY

**ALEX. J. WEDDERBURN**
SPECIAL AGENT

PUBLISHED BY ORDER OF CONGRESS
(Act approved August 8, 1894.)

WASHINGTON
GOVERNMENT PRINTING OFFICE
1894

# LETTER OF TRANSMITTAL.

U. S. DEPARTMENT OF AGRICULTURE,
DIVISION OF CHEMISTRY,
*Washington, D. C., May 10, 1894.*

SIR: I have the honor to present herewith the manuscript of a report prepared by Mr. A. J. Wedderburn, special agent, embracing a compilation of the pharmacy and drug laws of the several States and Territories.

Very respectfully,

H. W. WILEY,
*Chief.*

Hon. J. STERLING MORTON,
*Secretary.*

# LETTER OF SUBMITTAL.

U. S. DEPARTMENT OF AGRICULTURE,
DIVISION OF CHEMISTRY,
*Washington, D. C., June 14, 1893.*

SIR: I have the honor to submit herewith a complete copy of all pharmaceutical laws now in force in the several States and Territories and the District of Columbia.

There are no laws on this subject in the following States and Territories: Idaho, Indiana, Montana, Nevada, Arizona, and the Indian Territory. The Maryland law relates only to the city of Baltimore.

The thanks of the Department are due to the officers of the various State pharmaceutical associations for prompt compliance with requests for information, and it may not be out of place to add that these gentlemen, comprising a most important element of our population, almost unanimously evince great interest in the work undertaken by the Department in investigating adulteration, and seem anxious to see uniform laws enacted to prevent such practices.

Respectfully,

ALEX. J. WEDDERBURN,
*Special Agent.*

Dr. H. W. WILEY,
*Chemist.*

# CONTENTS.

|  | Page |
|---|---|
| Pharmacy and drug laws of the several States and Territories | 7 |
| Alabama | 7 |
| Arkansas | 10 |
| Arizona | 12 |
| California | 12 |
| Colorado | 16 |
| Connecticut | 20 |
| District of Columbia | 22 |
| Delaware | 25 |
| Florida | 27 |
| Georgia | 30 |
| Idaho | 34 |
| Illinois | 35 |
| Indiana | 38 |
| Indian Territory | 38 |
| Iowa | 38 |
| Kansas | 51 |
| Kentucky | 55 |
| Louisiana | 58 |
| Maine | 61 |
| Maryland | 62 |
| Massachusetts | 64 |
| Montana | 64 |
| Michigan | 66 |
| Minnesota | 69 |
| Mississippi | 75 |
| Missouri | 79 |
| Montana | 82 |
| Nebraska | 82 |
| Nevada | 85 |
| New Hampshire | 85 |
| New Jersey | 86 |
| New Mexico | 89 |
| New York | 91 |
| North Carolina | 95 |
| North Dakota | 99 |
| Oklahoma | 105 |
| Oregon | 108 |
| Ohio | 110 |
| Pennsylvania | 114 |
| Rhode Island | 118 |
| South Carolina | 121 |
| South Dakota | 124 |

|  | Page |
|---|---|
| Tennessee | 127 |
| Texas | 130 |
| Utah | 132 |
| Vermont | 135 |
| Virginia | 135 |
| Washington | 138 |
| West Virginia | 141 |
| Wisconsin | 144 |
| Wyoming | 148 |

# PHARMACY AND DRUG LAWS OF THE SEVERAL STATES AND TERRITORIES.

By ALEX. J. WEDDERBURN.

## ALABAMA.

### ALABAMA PHARMACY LAW.

AN ACT to regulate the practice of pharmacy and the sale of poisons in cities and towns of more than 900 inhabitants in the State of Alabama.

SEC. 1. *Be it enacted by the General Assembly of Alabama,* That from and after the passage of this act it shall be unlawful for any person not a registered pharmacist, within the meaning of this act, to conduct any pharmacy, drug store, apothecary shop, or store located in any village, town, or city in the State of Alabama of more than 900 inhabitants, or within two miles of any incorporated city or town of more than 900 inhabitants, for the purpose of retailing, compounding, or dispensing medicines or poisons for medical use, except as hereinafter provided.

SEC. 2. *Be it further enacted,* That it shall be unlawful for the proprietor of any store or pharmacy in any village, town, or city in the State of Alabama of more than 900 inhabitants, or within two miles of any incorporated city or town of more than 900 inhabitants, to allow any person except a registered pharmacist to compound or dispense the prescriptions of physicians, or to retail or dispense poisons for medical use, except as an aid to and under the supervision of a registered pharmacist. Any person violating the provisions of this section shall be deemed guilty of a misdemeanor, and on conviction shall be liable to a fine of not less than $25 nor more than $100 for each and every offense.

SEC. 3. *Be it further enacted,* That the governor shall appoint three persons from among the most prominent pharmacists in the State, all of whom shall have been residents of the State for five years, and at least five years' practical experience in their profession, who shall be known and styled "Board of Pharmacy for the State of Alabama," one of whom shall hold his office for one year, one for two years, and one for three years, and each until his successor shall be appointed and qualified; and each year thereafter another commissioner shall be so appointed for three years, and until a successor is appointed and qualified. If a vacancy occur in said board, another commissioner shall be appointed as aforesaid to fill the unexpired term thereof. Said board shall have power to make by-laws and all necessary regulations, and create auxiliary boards, if necessary, for the proper fulfillment of their duties under this act without expense to the State.

SEC. 4. *Be it further enacted,* That the board of pharmacy shall register in a suitable book the names and places of residence of all persons to whom they issue certificates, and date thereof. It shall be the duty of said board of pharmacy to register, without examination, as registered pharmacists, all pharmacists and druggists who are engaged in business in the State of Alabama, at the passage of this act, as owners or principals of stores or pharmacies in any village, town, or city of more than 900 inhabitants, for selling at retail, compounding or dispensing drugs, medicines, or chemicals for medical uses, or compounding or dispensing physicians' prescriptions, and all assistant pharmacists eighteen years of age engaged in said stores or pharmacies in any village, town, or city of more than 900 inhabitants in the State of Alabama, at the passage of this act, and who have been engaged as such in some store or pharmacy where physicians' prescriptions were compounded and dispensed: *Provided, however,* That in case of failure or neglect on the part of any person or persons to apply for registration within sixty days after they shall have been notified by said board of pharmacy for the State of Alabama, they shall undergo an examination as is provided for in section five of this act.

SEC. 5. *Be it further enacted,* That the said board of pharmacy shall, upon application, and at such time and place and in such manner as they may determine, either by a schedule of questions to be answered and subscribed to under oath, or orally, examine each and every person who shall desire to conduct the business of selling at retail, compounding or dispensing drugs, medicines, or chemicals for medicinal use, or compounding or dispensing physicians' prescriptions as pharmacists, and if a majority of said board shall be satisfied that said person is competent and fully qualified to conduct said business of compounding or dispensing drugs, medicines or chemicals for medicinal use, or to compound or dispense physicians' prescriptions, they shall enter the name of such person as a registered pharmacist in a book provided for in section four of this act; and that all graduates of colleges of pharmacy that require a practical experience in pharmacy of not less than four years before granting a diploma shall be entitled to have their names registered by said board without examination: *Provided, however,* That this act shall not be so construed as to prevent any physician who is authorized to practice medicine or surgery under the laws of this State from registering as a pharmacist or druggist, without examination: *Provided,* That any person or persons, not a pharmacist or druggist, may open and conduct such store if he or they keep constantly in their employ a registered pharmacist or druggist; but shall not himself or themselves sell or dispense drugs or medicines except proprietary and patent medicines in original packages.

SEC. 6. *Be it further enacted,* That the board of pharmacy shall be entitled to demand and receive of each person whom they register, and furnish a certificate as a registered pharmacist without examination, the sum of $2; and for each and every person that they examine orally, or whose answers to a schedule of questions are returned, subscribed to under oath, the sum of $3, which shall be in full for all services; and in case of examination of said person shall prove defective and unsatisfactory, and his name not to be registered, he shall be permitted to present himself for examination within any period not exceeding twelve months thereafter, and no charge shall be made for such examination.

SEC. 7. *Be it further enacted,* That every registered pharmacist, apothecary, and owner of any store shall be held responsible for the quality of all drugs, chemicals, or medicines he may sell or dispense, with the exception of those sold in original packages of the manufacturer and also those known as proprietary; and should he knowingly intermingle and fraudulently adulterate or cause to be adulterated such drugs, chemicals, or medical preparations, he shall be deemed guilty of a misdemeanor, and upon conviction thereof be liable to a penalty not exceeding $100, and in addition thereto his name shall be stricken from the register.

SEC. 8. *Be it further enacted,* That it shall be unlawful for any person, from and after the passage of this act, to retail any poison enumerated below: Arsenic and its preparations, corrosive sublimates, white and red precipitate, beniodide of mercury, cyanide of potassium, hydrocyanic acid, strychnine, and all poisonous vegetable alkaloids and their salts, and the essential oil of almonds; opium and its preparations, except paregoric and other preparations of opium containing less than two grains to the ounce; aconite, belladonna, colchicum, conium, nux vomica, henbane, savin, ergot, cotton root, cantharides, creosote, veratrum, digitalis, and their pharmaceutical preparations; croton oil, chloroform, chloral hydrate, sulphate of zinc, mineral acids, carbolic and oxalic acids, without labeling the box, vessel, or paper in which said poison is contained with the name of the article, the word poison, and the name and place of business of the seller. Nor shall it be lawful for any person to deliver or sell any poisons enumerated above unless, upon due inquiry, it be found that the purchaser is aware of its poisonous character and represents that it is to be used for a legitimate purpose. The provisions of this section shall not apply to the dispensing of poisons in not unusual quantities or doses upon the prescription of practitioners of medicine. Any violation of this section shall make the principal of said store liable to a fine of not less than $10 or more than $100, *Provided, however*, That this section shall not apply to manufacturers making and selling at wholesale any of the above poisons, and provided that each box, vessel, or paper in which said poison is contained shall be labeled with the name of the article, the word poison, and the name and place of business of the seller.

SEC. 9. *Be it further enacted*, That any itinerant vendor of any drug, poison, ointment, or appliance of any kind intended for treatment of any disease or injury, who shall, by writing or printing, or any other method, publicly profess to cure or treat disease or injury or deformity by any drug, nostrum, or manipulation, or other expedient, shall pay a license of $100 per annum to the State, to be paid in the manner for obtaining public license, or according to the usual laws in force for that purpose.

SEC. 10. *Be it further enacted*, That any person who shall procure or attempt to procure registration for himself or for another under this act, by making or causing to be made false representations, shall be deemed guilty of a misdemeanor, and shall, upon conviction thereof, be liable to a penalty of not less than $25 nor more than $100, and the name of the person so falsely registered shall be stricken from the register. Any person not a registered pharmacist as provided for in this act who shall conduct such a store, pharmacy, or place for retailing, compounding, or dispensing drugs, medicines, or chemicals, for medical use, or for compounding or dispensing physicians' prescriptions, or who shall take, use, or exhibit the title of registered pharmacist, shall be guilty of a misdemeanor, and upon conviction thereof shall be liable to a penalty of not less than $100.

SEC. 11. This act shall not apply to physicians putting up their own prescriptions.

SEC. 12. *Be it further enacted*, That it shall be the duty of every registered pharmacist to conspicuously post his certificate of registration in his place of business. Any person who shall fail to comply with all the provisions of this section shall be liable to a fine of $5 for each calendar month during which he is delinquent.

SEC. 13. The sum of $500 per year, or as much thereof as may be found necessary, is hereby appropriated, out of the money so received for license, for the expense of said board of pharmacy. All surplus over and above such amount to be divided as follows: One-half to the Pharmaceutical Association, the remainder to be paid into the State treasury.

SEC. 14. All suits for recovery of the several penalties prescribed in this act shall be presented in the name of the State of Alabama in any court having jurisdiction, and it shall be the duty of the State's attorney of the county wherein such offense is committed to present all persons violating the provisions of this act upon proper complaint being made.

SEC. 15. *Be it further enacted*, That all laws and parts of laws in conflict with the provisions of this act be, and the same are hereby, repealed.

Approved February 28, 1887.

# ARKANSAS.

## The Arkansas Pharmacy Law.

A BILL for an act to be entitled an act to establish the Arkansas State Board of Pharmacy, and to prescribe the powers and duties of said board, and to regulate the compounding and vending of medicines, drugs, and poisons in the State of Arkansas, and to provide a penalty for the infringement of the act.

### PREAMBLE.

Whereas in all civilized countries it has been found necessary to regulate the traffic in medicines and poisons, and to provide by law for the regulation of the delicate and responsible business of compounding and dispensing the powerful agents used in medicines; and

Whereas the safety and welfare of the public are endangered by the sale of poisons by unqualified and ignorant persons; and

Whereas the power of physicians to overcome disease depends greatly upon their ability to procure good, unadulterated drugs and skillfully prepared medicines; and

Whereas the sophistication and adulteration of drugs and medicines is a specious fraud which should be prevented and suitably punished: Therefore,

*Be it enacted by the General Assembly of the State of Arkansas:* SEC. 1. That from and after the passage of this act it shall be unlawful for any person not a registered pharmacist, within the meaning of this act, to conduct any drug store, pharmacy or apothecary shop, or store for the purpose of retailing, compounding, or dispensing medicines in any city or incorporated town in the State of Arkansas, except as hereinafter provided, and that it shall be unlawful for the proprietor of such store or pharmacy to allow any person other than a registered pharmacist to compound or dispense the prescriptions of physicians, except as an aid to and under the supervision of a registered pharmacist. Any person violating the provisions of this section shall be deemed guilty of a misdemeanor, and, on conviction thereof, shall be liable to a fine of not less than five or more than one hundred dollars.

SEC. 2. That within sixty days after the passage of this act the governor shall appoint five experienced pharmacists, who shall have been actively engaged in the drug business for the last five years immediately preceding their appointment, who shall constitute the Arkansas State Board of Pharmacy, one of whom shall hold his office for one year, one for two years, one for three years, one for four years, and one for five years, and each until his successor shall have been appointed and qualified, which terms shall be decided by lot at the time of organization. And annually thereafter the governor shall appoint one member of said board, with qualifications as above set forth, who shall hold his office for five years and until his successor is appointed and qualified. In case of a vacancy from death or other cause, the governor shall appoint a successor, with qualifications as above set forth.

SEC. 3. That before entering upon the duties of said office, the members of the said board shall take the oath prescribed by the constitution of the State for State officers, and shall file the same in the office of the secretary of State, who shall thereupon issue to each of the said examiners a certificate of appointment.

SEC. 4. That immediately after the appointment and qualification of the board they shall meet and organize as a State board of pharmacy by electing from their own number a president and secretary. The board may adopt such by-laws, rules, and regulations as they may deem necessary to carry into execution the provisions of this act without expense to the State. A majority of the board shall be a quorum for the transaction of any business.

SEC. 5. The board of pharmacy shall hold not less than two stated regular meetings per annum for the examination of candidates, one of which may be held at the time and place of the annual meeting of the Arkansas Association of Pharmacists, and the other meeting shall be held at such time and place as the board may determine. Other meetings of the board may also be held whenever and wherever a quorum of the board, including the secretary, is present. In the interim of the sessions of the board, and upon satisfactory evidence of the fitness of the applicant, any member of the board may, in his discretion, issue a temporary certificate, which shall authorize and empower the holder to conduct a drug store or pharmacy, as set forth in section 1 of this act. Such temporary certificate shall terminate and expire at the date of the next succeeding regular meeting of the board after the granting thereof. A fee of $2 shall be demanded for this temporary certificate, which shall be part payment of the regular examination fee as hereinafter set forth.

SEC. 6. The board of pharmacy shall register in a suitable book the names and places of residence of all persons to whom they issue certificates, and the dates thereof. Upon written application, accompanied by such reasonable evidence as the board may require, it shall be the duty of said board of pharmacy to register, without examination, as registered pharmacists, all druggists and pharmacists who are engaged in the business in any city or incorporated town in the State of Arkansas at the passage of this act, either as owners, managers, or clerks of any drug store, pharmacy, or apothecary shop: *Provided*, That no druggist's clerk shall be so registered unless he be 18 years of age and has been engaged for the space of three years next preceding the passage of this act in some drug store or pharmacy where physicians' prescriptions were compounded.

In case of the failure or neglect of any person to apply for registration within sixty days after the organization of the board of pharmacy, and publication thereof in the weekly paper published in the State of Arkansas whose circulation is the largest of all the papers so published, such person shall have forfeited the privilege of being registered as a registered pharmacist as set forth in this section.

SEC. 7. The State board of pharmacy shall, upon application, and at such time and place, in such manner as they may determine, examine every person who shall desire to conduct the business described in section 1 of this act in any city or incorporated town in the State of Arkansas; and if a majority of the members present at the meeting of the board shall be satisfied that said person is competent and fully qualified to conduct the said business of compounding and dispensing drugs, medicines, or chemicals for medical use, the board shall enter the name of such person as a registered pharmacist in the book provided for in section 6 of this act: *Provided*, That all graduates in pharmacy of schools or colleges of pharmacy that require three years' practical experience before granting diplomas shall be entitled to have their names registered as registered pharmacists by the board of pharmacy without examination. The board of pharmacy shall issue an appropriate certificate to each person registered, which certificate must be conspicuously displayed in every store described in this act.

SEC. 8. The board of pharmacy shall be entitled to demand and receive from each person whom they register as a registered pharmacist, without examination, the sum of $3, and from each and every person whom they examine the sum of $6, which shall be in full for the registration and the certificate. In case the examination of said person proves defective and unsatisfactory to the board, and he being declined registration, he shall have the privilege of reëxamination within twelve months thereafter, without any fee being charged him.

SEC. 9. Any registered pharmacist who shall knowingly, intentionally, and fraudulently adulterate, or cause to be adulterated, any drugs, chemicals, or medical preparations, and offer such adulterations for sale, shall be deemed guilty of a misdemeanor, and, upon conviction therefor, his license shall thereby be revoked, and, in addition thereto, he shall be liable to a penalty of not less than $5 nor more than $100.

SEC. 10. If any person shall procure registration as a registered pharmacist under this act by making, or causing to be made, false representations, the registration and certificate thus fraudulently obtained may, in the discretion of the board, be revoked, and the name of the person so registered stricken from the register: *Pro-*

*vided,* That the person charged with the fraud be first allowed a hearing by the board.

SEC. 11. Any person not a registered pharmacist, as provided in this act, who shall conduct a drug store or pharmacy, or place for compounding or dispensing drugs, medicines, or chemicals for medicinal use, in any city or incorporated town in the State of Arkansas, or who shall take, use, or exhibit the title of registered pharmacist without the same has been regularly conferred on him, as set forth in sections 6 and 7 of this act, shall be deemed guilty of a misdemeanor, and upon conviction therefor [thereof] be liable to a penalty of not less than $5 nor more than $100: *Provided,* That any person or persons, not a registered pharmacist, may own or conduct such a store, if he or they keep constantly in their store a registered pharmacist: *Provided further,* That this act shall not apply to physicians putting up their own prescriptions, nor to the sale of those articles commonly known as "grocers' drugs," nor to the sale of patent or proprietary medicines or non-secret medicines.

SEC. 12. If any registered pharmacist shall be convicted by a court of competent jurisdiction, in this State, of the illegal sale or handling of intoxicating liquors his certificate as registered pharmacist shall thereupon become null and void, and his license or authority to engage in the business, as set forth in section 1 of this act, shall be thereupon revoked.

SEC. 13. If any registered pharmacist shall go out of the drug business and remain out for a period of twelve months, his certificate as a registered pharmacist shall thereupon expire.

SEC. 14. All suits for the recovery of the several penalties prescribed in this act shall be prosecuted in the name of the State of Arkansas, in any court having jurisdiction, and it shall be the duty of the prosecuting attorney of the county where such offense is committed to prosecute all persons violating the provisions of this act upon proper complaint being made. All penalties collected under the provisions of this act shall inure to the public-school fund of the school district in which the offense was committed.

SEC. 15. Nothing in this act shall be construed to repeal or in any wise interfere with the collection of the "privilege taxes" now levied, for State, county, or city purposes, on the business of hawking, peddling, or street vending of goods, wares, and merchandise.

SEC. 16. All persons registered under this act shall be exempt and free from jury duty in the State of Arkansas.

SEC. 17. All acts and parts of acts in conflict with this act be, and the same are hereby repealed, and this act shall take effect and be in force from and after its passage.

## ARIZONA.

Governor L. C. Hughes, under date June 1, 1893, says the State of Arizona has no pharmacy law.

## CALIFORNIA.

### CHAPTER 85.

AN ACT to regulate the practice of pharmacy and sale of poisons in the State of California.

*The People of the State of California, represented in Senate and Assembly, do enact as follows:*

SECTION 1. From and after the first day of January, A. D. eighteen hundred and ninety-two, it shall be unlawful for any person to conduct any pharmacy or store for dispensing or compounding medicines, unless such person be a registered pharmacist, within the meaning of this act; and it shall be unlawful for any person to compound or dispense any physician's prescription, unless such person be a registered pharmacist, or a registered assistant pharmacist, within the meaning of this act, except as hereinafter provided.

SEC. 2. Any person in order to be a registered pharmacist, must be a graduate of pharmacy, a licentiate in pharmacy, or a practicing pharmacist.

SEC. 3. Graduates in pharmacy are persons who have had four years' experience in stores where the prescriptions of medical practitioners are compounded, and each must have obtained a diploma from a legally constituted college of pharmacy. Licentiates in pharmacy are persons who have had four years' experience in stores where the prescriptions of medical practitioners are compounded, and shall have passed an examination before the State board of pharmacy, or who shall present satisfactory credentials or certificates of their attainments to the said board. Practicing pharmacists are persons who, at the passage of this act, are conducting pharmacies in this State for compounding and dispensing of prescriptions of medical practitioners, and for the sale of medicines and poisons. Assistant pharmacists are persons of not less than eighteen years of age, who are employed by registered pharmacists, have studied the art of pharmacy for two years, and have passed an examination by the board of pharmacy, or who, prior to the passage of this act, have had three years' experience in pharmacies.

SEC. 4. Every pharmacist claiming the right of registration under this act shall, on or before the first day of January next after its passage, forward to the board of pharmacy satisfactory proof that he was engaged in the business of preparing and dispensing medicines and physicians' prescriptions at the time of passage of this act, or that he is otherwise entitled to registration under its provisions. The board of pharmacy shall then issue to said applicant, upon his paying the sum of five dollars, a certificate of registration. Any practicing pharmacist failing to comply with the requirements of this section, within sixty days from and after the first day of January, eighteen hundred and ninety-two, shall forfeit his right to registration, and shall appear for examination, as provided for in this act.

SEC. 5. Every assistant pharmacist claiming right of registration under this act, without passing an examination by the board of pharmacy, shall, on or before the first day of January next after the passage, forward to the board of pharmacy satisfactory proof that he has had three years' experience in drug stores where physicians' prescriptions are prepared; the board of pharmacy shall then issue to said applicant, upon his paying the sum of one dollar, a certificate of registration as assistant pharmacist. Any assistant failing to comply with the requirements of this section, within sixty days from and after the first day of January, eighteen hundred and ninety-two, shall forfeit his right to registration without passing the examination provided for in this act. No registered assistant shall conduct a pharmacy, or be granted a certificate as a registered pharmacist, until he has passed the examination for licentiate in pharmacy, as required by this act.

SEC. 6. Within thirty days after the passage of this act, and every fourth year thereafter, the governor shall appoint seven competent pharmacists, residing in different parts of the State, to serve as a board of pharmacy. The members of this board shall, within thirty days after their appointment, individually take and subscribe, before the county clerk in the county in which they individually reside, on oath, faithfully and impartially to discharge the duties prescribed by this act. They shall hold office for the term of four years, and until their successors are appointed and qualified. In case of vacancy in the board of pharmacy, the governor shall fill the same by appointing a member to serve for the remainder of the term only. The office of said board shall be located in San Francisco. The board shall organize by electing a president and a secretary, the latter to be ex-officio treasurer of the board. Four members of the board shall constitute a quorum. They shall meet at least quarterly, and have the power to make by-laws for the proper fulfillment of their duties. The duties of the board shall be to transact all business pertaining to the legal regulations of the practice of pharmacy; to investigate all complaints respecting noncompliance with, or violation of, the provisions of this act, and to bring the same to the notice of the proper prosecuting officer, whenever there appears to the board to be reasonable grounds for such action, and to examine and register as pharmacists, or assistant pharmacists, all applicants whom it shall deem qualified to be such, respectively. All persons, on applying for examination or registration, shall pay to the secretary a fee of five dollars for licentiate, and two dollars for assistants; and on passing the examination shall be furnished with a certificate, signed by the secretary and examiners. In case of failure to pass, the board shall grant a second examination within one year, without any additional fee being charged. The board shall render an annual report of its proceedings to the governor of the State.\*

Sec. 7. It shall be the duty of the secretary to keep a book of registration open at the city of San Francisco, of which due notice shall be given through the public press or by mail, in which book shall be entered, under the supervision of the board, the names, titles, qualifications, and places of business of all persons coming under the provisions of this act. The secretary shall give receipts for all money received by him, and disburse the same by order of the board for necessary expenses, taking proper vouchers therefor. The balance of said moneys, after paying the expenses of the board, he shall pay to the State treasurer, who shall keep it as a special fund to be used in carrying out the provisions of this act.

Sec. 8. The members of the board of pharmacy shall each be paid the sum of five dollars per diem, for every meeting of the board which they attend, and the secretary shall receive such additional compensation as the board may direct. All compensation of members, and other expenses of the board of pharmacy, shall be paid out of the examination and registration fees and fines.

Sec. 9. No person shall add to or remove from, or cause to be added to or removed from, any drug, chemical, or medicinal preparation, any ingredient or material for the purpose of adulteration or substitution, or which shall deteriorate the quality, commercial value, or medicinal effect, or alter the nature or composition of such article; and no person shall knowingly sell, or offer for sale, any such adulterated, altered, or substituted drug, chemical, or medicinal preparation, without informing the purchaser of the adulteration or sophistication of the article sold or offered for sale. Every registered pharmacist shall file or cause to be filed all physicians' prescriptions compounded or dispensed in his pharmacy or store; they shall be preserved for two years, and he shall furnish a correct copy of any prescription, upon the order or request of the attending physician. Any person who shall willfully violate any of the provisions of this section shall be guilty of a misdemeanor, and upon conviction thereof shall be liable to all costs of the action; and for the first offense be liable to a fine not exceeding fifty dollars, and for each subsequent offense a fine of not less than fifty nor more than one hundred dollars, said fines to be paid over to the board of pharmacy. On written complaint being entered against any person or persons, charging them with specific violation of any of the provisions of this act, the board of pharmacy is hereby empowered to delegate one of its members, or other suitable person, who shall have authority to inspect drugs, chemicals, or medicines, and to make a thorough investigation of the case; he shall then report the result of his investigation, and if such report justify such action, the board shall notify the prosecuting attorney or district attorney, who shall prosecute the offender according to law.

Sec. 10. It shall be unlawful for any person to retail any poisons enumerated in schedules "A" and "B," appended to this act, without labelling the box, bottle, or paper in which said poison is contained, with the name of the article, the word "Poison," and the name and place of business of the seller. Nor shall it be lawful to sell or deliver any poison named in schedules "A" and "B," unless, on inquiry, it is found that the person is aware of its poisonous character, and that it is to be used for a legitimate purpose. Nor shall it be lawful to sell or deliver any poison included in schedule "A" without making, or causing to be made, an entry in a book kept for that purpose only, stating the date of sale, and the name and

---

\* See amendment at end of this law.

address of the purchaser, the name and quantity of the poison sold, the purpose for which it is stated by the purchaser to be required, and the name of the dispenser; said book to always be open for inspection by the proper authorities, and to be preserved for at least five years. The provisions of this section shall not apply to the dispensing of poisons when prescribed by practitioners of medicine, nor to the sale of poisons, if a single bottle or package does not contain more than an ordinary dose. Dealers shall affix to every bottle, box, parcel or other inclosure of an original package containing any of the articles named in schedules "A" and "B" of this act, a suitable label or brand with the word "Poison," but they are hereby exempted from the registration of the sale of such articles when sold at wholesale, or to a registered pharmacist or physician. Any person failing to comply with the requirements of this section shall be guilty of misdemeanor, and upon conviction shall be liable to a fine not exceeding fifty dollars.

SEC. 11. Any person who shall attempt to procure registration for himself, or for any other person under this act, by making, or causing to be made, any false representations, or who shall fraudulently represent himself to be registered, shall be deemed guilty of a misdemeanor, and shall, upon conviction thereof, be fined in a sum not exceeding two hundred dollars. Any registered pharmacist who shall permit the compounding and dispensing of prescriptions of medical practitioners in his store by persons not registered, except by junior assistants under the direct supervision of registered persons, or any person not registered who shall retail medicines or poisons, except in a pharmacy under the supervision of a registered pharmacist or a registered assistant pharmacist, and any registered person who shall fail to comply with the regulations of this act, shall be guilty of a misdemeanor, and upon conviction thereof be fined not exceeding fifty dollars. Nothing in this act shall apply to or interfere with the business of any practitioner of medicine who does not keep a pharmacy or open shop for the retailing of medicines or poisons, nor with the exclusive wholesale business of any dealer, except that portion of section ten which relates to marking or labeling certain poisons mentioned in this Act. Nor shall general dealers come under the provisions of this act, in so far as it relates to the keeping for sale of proprietary medicines in original packages of drugs and medicines; but in no case shall they compound or prepare any pharmaceutical preparations or prescriptions.

SEC. 12. All persons registered under this act shall be exempt and free from jury duty.

### SCHEDULE "A."

Arsenic, corrosive sublimate, cynanide of potassium, hydrocyanic acid, strichnia, cocaine, and all other poisonous vegetable alkaloids and their salts, opium, and all its preparations, excepting those which contain less than two grains to the ounce.

### SCHEDULE "B."

Aconite, belladonna, colchicum, conium, nux vomica, savin, cantharides, phosphorus, digitalis, and their pharmaceutical preparations, croton oil, chloroform, chloral, sulphate of zinc, sugar of lead, mineral acids, carbolic acid, and oxalic acid, white precipitate, red precipitate, biniodide of mercury, essential oil of almonds.

All acts or parts of acts which conflict with this are hereby repealed.

Approved, March 11, 1891.

### CHAPTER LVII.

AN ACT to amend an act entitled "An act to regulate the practice of pharmacy and sale of poisons in the State of California," approved March 11, 1891.

*The People of the State of California, represented in Senate and Assembly, do enact as follows:*

SECTION 1. Section six of said act is hereby amended so as to read as follows:

SEC. 6. Within thirty days after the passage of this act, and every fourth year thereafter, the governor shall appoint seven competent pharmacists, residing in different parts of the State, to serve as a board of pharmacy. The members of this board shall, within thirty days after their appointment, individually take and subscribe, before the county clerk in the county in which they individually reside, an oath faithfully and impartially to discharge the duties prescribed by this act. They shall hold office for the term of four years, and until their successors are appointed and qualified. In case of vacancy in the board of pharmacy, the governor shall fill the same by appointing a member to serve for the remainder of the term only. The office of said board shall be located in San Francisco. The board shall organize by electing a president and a secretary, the latter to be ex officio treasurer of the board. Four members of the board shall constitute a quorum. They shall meet at least quarterly, and have power to make by-laws for the proper fulfillment of their duties. The duties of the board shall be to transact all business pertaining to the legal regulations of the practice of pharmacy; to investigate all complaints repecting non-compliance with or violations of the provisions of this act, and to bring the same to the notice of the proper prosecuting officer, whenever there appears to the board to be reasonable grounds for such action; and to examine and register as pharmacists, or assistant pharmacists, all applicants whom it shall deem qualified to be such, respectively. All persons, on applying for examination or registration, shall pay to the secretary a fee of five dollars for licentiate, and two dollars for assistants; and on passing the examination they shall be furnished with a certificate signed by the secretary and examiners. In case of failure to pass, the board shall grant a second examination within one year without any additional fee being charged. Every registered pharmacist who desires to continue the practice of his profession in this State shall, annually, on such date as the board of pharmacy may determine, pay to the secretary of the said board a registration fee, to be fixed by the board, but which shall in no case exceed the sum of two dollars per annum, for which he shall receive a renewal of said registration. Every registered assistant pharmacist who desires to continue the practice of his profession in this State shall, annually, on such date as the board of pharmacy may determine, pay to the secretary of said board a registration fee, to be fixed by the board, but which shall in no case exceed the sum of one dollar per annum, for which he shall receive a renewal of said registration. The board shall render an annual report of its proceedings to the governor of the State.

Approved, March 3, 1893.

## COLORADO.

AN ACT in relation to the practice of pharmacy and the sale of medicines and poisons; licensing persons to carry on such practice, and exempting them from jury duty; providing for the appointment and prescribing the powers and duties of a state board of pharmacy; and to repeal an act entitled "An act regulating the practice of pharmacy; licensing persons to carry on such practice and exempting them from jury duty; providing for the appointment and prescribing the powers and duties of a board of pharmacists."

*Be it enacted by the General Assembly of the State of Colorado:*

SECTION 1. That it shall hereafter be unlawful for any person other than a registered or assistant pharmacist, as hereinafter defined, to retail, compound, or dispense drugs, medicines or pharmacal preparations in the State of Colorado; or to institute, conduct, or manage a pharmacy, store, or shop for the retailing, compounding, or dispensing of drugs, medicines, or pharmacal preparations in said State of Colorado, unless such person shall be a registered pharmacist, as this act provides, or shall place in charge of said pharmacy, store, or shop, a registered pharmacist, except as hereinafter provided.

SEC. 2. "*Registered pharmacists*" shall comprise all persons regularly registered as such in the State of Colorado for the year ending July 2, 1893; and all other persons registered as licentiates in pharmacy for the aforesaid period who have been authorized to conduct or manage a pharmacy in the State of Colorado; and all persons over twenty-one years of age, having four years' practical experience in compounding and dispensing of physicians' prescriptions, who shall pass a satisfactory examination before the State board of pharmacy. Graduates in pharmacy who have obtained diplomas from such colleges and shools of pharmacy as shall be approved by the board of pharmacy, and who, previous to obtaining said diploma, have had four years' experience in the dispensing of physicians' prescriptions, *may*, on payment of a fee of $5, be made registered pharmacists.

SEC. 3. "*Assistant pharmacists,*" in the meaning of this act, shall comprise all persons regularly registered as licentiates in pharmacy in the State of Colorado for the year ending July 2, 1893, who have been authorized to "assist in the dispensing and compounding of physicians' prescriptions," under the supervision of a properly qualified person; and all persons over eighteen years of age, having two years' practical experience in the compounding and dispensing of physicians' prescriptions, who shall pass such examination as the State board of pharmacy shall require. Assistant pharmacists shall not be permitted to conduct or manage a pharmacy on their own account, nor assume the management of such business for others.

SEC. 4. Immediately upon the passage of this act, and biennially thereafter, the Colorado Pharmacal Association may submit to the governor of the State of Colorado, the names of ten or more registered pharmacists having at least ten years' experience as dispensing pharmacists; and from this number the governor shall appoint three; and the said three registered pharmacists shall constitute the State board of pharmacy of the State of Colorado, to have and to hold office for the term of two years, or until their successors shall have been duly appointed and qualified.

In case of resignation or removal from the State of any member of said board, or of a vacancy occurring from any cause, the governor shall appoint a registered pharmacist to serve as a member of the board for the remainder of the unexpired term.

SEC. 5. The said board shall, within thirty days after its appointment, meet in the city of Denver, and organize by the selection of a president, secretary, and treasurer, who shall serve for the term of one year, and who shall perform the duties prescribed by the board. Meetings for the examination of applicants for registration, granting of certificates, and the transaction of such other necessary business, shall be held at least once in four months, and at such times and places as may be fixed upon by the board: *Provided,* That ten days' public notice of the time and place of each meeting at which there is an examination of candidates for registration shall be given.

It shall be the duty of the board to receive all applications for examination and registration submitted in proper form, to grant certificates to such persons as may be entitled to the same under this act; to cause the prosecution of all persons violating any of the provisions of this act; to report annually to the governor and to the State Pharmacal Association, upon the condition of pharmacy in the State of Colorado, which report shall furnish also a record of the proceedings of the board, as well as the names of all persons registered under this act; to keep a book for registration in which shall be entered the names and places of business of all persons registered under this act; on what grounds, and under which particular section of this act each was registered, and any other facts pertaining to the granting of certificates.

The board shall have power to make by-laws for the full and proper execution of its duties under this act; to prescribe the forms and methods of application, examination and registration; to demand and receive from applicants the fees herein provided, which shall be held by the board and applied to the payment of salaries and other necessary expenses incident to the full discharge of its duties.

SEC. 6. The salaries of said board shall be $5.00 to each member for each day of actual service, and all legitimate expenses incurred in the discharge of official duties.

The secretary of said board shall receive an additional salary, to be fixed by the board, and not to exceed $500.00 per annum; he shall pay to the treasurer at each regular meeting, or whenever the board may direct, such funds of the board as may be in his possession, and take the treasurer's receipt therefor: *Provided*, That no part of the salaries or expenses of the board shall be paid out of the State treasury.

In its annual reports to the governor and the Colorado Pharmaceutical Association the board shall render an account of all moneys received and disbursed, pursuant to this act; and the secretary and treasurer shall give such bonds as said board shall from time to time direct.

SEC. 7. Every person seeking registration under this act whose registration is not otherwise provided for, shall make application in form and manner prescribed by the board, and deposit with the secretary of the board a fee of $5.00; then on presenting himself at the time and place directed by the board, and sustaining a satisfactory examination, he shall be granted an appropriate certificate, setting forth his particular qualifications: *Provided*, That in case of failure of an applicant to pass a satisfactory examination, he shall be entitled to a second examination, without charge at the next succeeding meeting of the board.

SEC. 8. Every registered pharmacist, and every assistant pharmacist, in the meaning of this act, who desires to continue in the pursuit of pharmacy in this State, shall annually, after the expiration of the first year of registration, and on or before the 2nd day of July of each year, pay to the secretary of the board of pharmacy a renewal fee, to be fixed by the board, but which shall not exceed $2, in return for which a renewal of registration shall be issued. If any person shall fail or neglect to procure his annual registration as herein specified, notice of such failure having been mailed to his post-office address, as obtained from the books of the secretary, the board may, after the expiration of thirty days following the issue of said notice, deprive him of his registration and all other privileges conferred by this act; in order to gain registration it shall be necessary for such persons to make application and pass examination as provided in section 7 of this act.

SEC. 9. Every person registered under this act shall receive from the State board an appropriate certificate, not exceeding in size 120 square inches, which shall be conspicuously displayed at all times in his place of business. If the holder be entitled to manage or conduct a pharmacy in this State for himself or another, the fact shall be set forth in the certificate.

SEC. 10. Any person who is not a registered pharmacist, in the meaning of this act, who shall keep a pharmacy, store, or shop for the compounding and dispensing of physicians' prescriptions, and who shall not have in his employ in said pharmacy, store, or shop a registered pharmacist, in the meaning of this act, shall for each and every such offense be liable to a fine of $250.

SEC. 11. Any person who shall unlawfully and without authority under this act, take, use, or exhibit the title of registered pharmacist or assistant pharmacist in the State of Colorado, shall be liable to a fine of $100 for each and every such offense; a like penalty shall attach to any assistant pharmacist who shall, without authority, take, use, or exhibit the title of registered pharmacist in the State of Colorado.

SEC. 12. Any proprietor of a pharmacy, or other person, who shall permit the compounding and dispensing of physicians' prescriptions, or the vending of drugs, medicines, or pharmacal preparations in his store or place of business, except by a registered pharmacist, or assistant pharmacist, in the meaning of this act, or under the immediate supervision of one, or who, while continuing in the pursuit of pharmacy in the State of Colorado, shall fail or neglect to procure his annual registration, or any person who shall willfully make any false representations to procure for himself or for another registration under this act, or who shall violate any other provision of this act, shall for each and every offense be liable to a fine of $100: *Provided*, That nothing in this act shall interfere with the business of those merchants who keep on sale such poisons, acids, and chemicals as are regularly used in agriculture, mining, and the arts, when kept and sold for such purposes only in sealed and plainly labeled packages: *Provided, also*, That nothing in this act shall in any manner interfere with the business of any physician in regular practice, nor prevent him from supplying to his patients such articles as may to him seem proper, nor with the marketing and vending of proprietary and patent medicines, nor with the exclusive wholesale business of any dealers, except as hereinafter provided: *Provided, also,* That nothing in this act shall in any manner interfere with the business of merchants in towns having less than 500 inhabitants, in which there is no licensed pharmacy, to sell or vend such medicines, compounds, and chemicals as are required by the general public, and in form and manner prescibed by the board of pharmacy.

SEC. 13. The proprietors of establishments other than pharmacies, and where physicians' prescriptions are not dispensed, as well as itinerant vendors of merchandise, shall not be permitted to sell, keep on sale, or give away any of the articles mentioned or included in schedule A of this act; nor any patent or proprietary preparation for medicinal, dietetic, or toilet purposes known to contain in large or small proportion any of such ingredients; nor any other chemical or pharmacal compound the use of which, for a short or long period of time, might be attended with injury to health or morals, unless the container of said preparation, or the wrapper enclosing it, shall have affixed a "caution" label such as the board of pharmacy shall devise and direct. It shall be the duty of the board, when called upon, to furnish dealers with a list of such articles, preparations, and compounds the sale of which is prohibited or regulated by this section. Any person violating any of the provisions of this section, or evading any of the requirements herein imposed, or authorizing the same to be done by another, shall be liable to a fine of not less than $100 nor more than $500 for each and every offense; and any person who shall willfully make any false representation about the character or composition of any preparation or compound, with the object of deceiving the officers of the State, or defeating the purposes of this act, shall, for every such offense, be liable to a fine of not less than $100 or imprisonment in the county jail for not less than thirty days, or both. All suits brought on account of violations of any of the provisions of this act shall be prosecuted in the name of the people of Colorado, in any court of competent jurisdiction; and it shall be the duty of the district attorney where the offense is committed to prosecute every person violating any provision of this act upon proper complaint being made. All fines or penalties collected for such violation shall be paid to the State board of pharmacy, to be held by said board as by this act required.

SEC. 14. All persons registered under the provisions of this act, and actively engaged in the practice of pharmacy, shall be exempt from serving as jurors.

SEC. 15. Annually on the first day of July of each year, the State board of pharmacy shall pay into the treasury of the Colorado State Pharmacal Association all moneys then held by said board over and above the sum of $300, and which have been received by said board as penalties for violations of this act, or as registration fees for the expiring year: *Provided,* That the moneys thus paid to the State Pharmacal Association shall be held by said association as a fund for educational and scientific purposes.

SEC. 16. An act entitled "An act regulating the practice of pharmacy, licensing persons to carry on such practice, and exempting them from jury duty; providing for the appointment, and prescribing the powers and duties, of a board of pharmacists," approved April 2, 1887, and all acts and parts of acts in conflict with the provisions of this act, are hereby repealed.

SEC. 17. Inasmuch as an emergency exists, this act shall be in force from and after its passage.

SCHEDULE A.

Aconite, belladonna, conium, henbane, nux vomica, opium, ergot, cantharides, digitalis, and ipecacuanha and their preparations, alkaloids and other derivatives.

Morphine, strychnine, codeine, cocaine and all other alkaloids and their salts.

Chloral, chloroform, ether, oil of tansy, oil pennyroyal, and all other hypnotics, ecbolics and emmenagogue agents.

Mercury, copper, antimony, zinc, iron, lead, gold, arsenic, and silver, their salts and compounds. All cyanides, iodides, bromides.

# CONNECTICUT.

## Pharmacy Act.

[Title LV, General Statutes, 1888. Chapter CLXXXVIII.]

### AN ACT relating to medicines and poisons.

*Be it enacted by the Senate and House of Representatives in General Assembly convened:*

SECTION 3118. There shall be three commissioners of pharmacy, consisting of one reputable physician and two pharmacists, to be selected by the governor from six persons to be annually nominated to him by the Connecticut Pharmaceutical Association.

SEC. 3119. The governor shall, on or before the first day of June in the year eighteen hundred and eighty-eight, and annually thereafter, appoint one such commissioner, who shall hold office for three years from the first day of June in the year of his appointment; and vacancies may be filled by the governor for the unexpired portion of the term.

SEC. 3120. Said commissioners shall keep a record of their proceedings, and may give certified copies thereof, which shall be legal evidence.

SEC. 3121. No person shall conduct or keep a shop, store, or place of any kind for retailing drugs, medicines, poisons, or such chemicals as are used in compounding medicines, or compound or dispense prescriptions of a physician, or vend medicines or poisons, unless he shall have been licensed therefor, as hereinafter provided, or shall be under the supervision of a licensed pharmacist.

SEC. 3122. The comptroller shall designate a room in the capitol for the meeting of said commissioners, which shall be held in each year on the first Tuesdays of March, April, June, September, and December, and at such other times and places as they may deem necessary, to determine the qualifications of applicants for license as pharmacists, and said commissioners shall license, by a certificate signed by them, or by a majority of them, such persons as shall produce satisfactory evidence to them of their qualifications and attainments, either by diploma granted to the applicant by some reputable college of pharmacy, or by the certificate of some reputable pharmacist that the applicant has, for not less than three years prior to his application, received instruction in pharmacy and possesses the necessary qualifications of a pharmacist, or by other satisfactory evidence.

SEC. 3123. All applicants for a license, other than a renewal of a license previously granted by said commissioners, shall be personally examined by said commissioners: *Provided, however,* That such examinations may be omitted in the cases of applicants who exhibit to said commissioners a diploma granted by some reputable college of pharmacy, or a license in force within one year prior to the date of such application, granted by the board of commissioners of pharmacy of another State, if such license shall be deemed sufficient evidence of qualifications by the commissioners of pharmacy of this State. Licenses shall specify the name of the person licensed, the date when granted, the city or town in which he shall conduct his business; and if in a city, the street and number of his place of business; and his license shall be conspicuously exhibited in his place of business, and shall remain in force until the first day of April next after said date, unless granted at a meeting of said commissioners on the first Tuesday of March, in which case such license shall terminate on the thirty-first day of March of the succeeding year, or unless such person shall remove his place of business without notice to the commissioners; and a license may be renewed upon the application of the person licensed, upon the terms hereinafter provided.

SEC. 3124. Every person conducting the business of pharmacy shall, on or before the first Tuesday of March annually, apply to said commissioners for said license, or for a renewal thereof, and establish his right thereto by such evidence as shall be satisfactory to them; and they shall adopt forms for application for license, and rules and regulations prescribing the manner in which the evidence in support of such application shall be presented to them; and they shall furnish such forms and such rules and regulations to any person upon his request.

SEC. 3125. Each applicant shall pay to said commissioners three dollars for his license and two dollars for each renewal thereof; and whenever a personal examination shall be made as provided in the preceding section, a fee of five dollars; but if upon such examination a license shall be refused, said fee shall be refunded to said applicant; but if any such applicant shall make a new application, and a license shall be again refused, said fee shall not in that case be refunded. And said commissioners shall account semiannually, on the first Tuesdays of December and June, with the treasurer of the State, for the sums received by them for licenses, and shall be paid by the State at the time of such accounting, the money necessarily expended by them for stationery and printing, and compensation for their services at the rate of three hundred dollars per annum to each commissioner: *Provided*, That if the amounts received by said commissioners for said licenses shall not be sufficient to pay them said sums for services in full, such amounts shall be apportioned *pro rata* among said commissioners, and their charges for expenses for stationery and printing, and for services, shall be audited and approved by the comptroller in the proportion aforesaid, who shall draw his order upon the treasury therefor.

SEC. 3126. Nothing contained in the preceding sections of this chapter shall be construed to prevent a practicing physician from compounding his own prescriptions, or to prevent the sale of proprietary medicines, or of any drugs, medicines, or poisons, at wholesale to licensed pharmacists, or for use in manufactures or the arts, or to prevent any person from becoming a partner in or the proprietor of a pharmacy conducted by a licensed pharmacist, or any keeper of a country store from keeping for sale and selling such domestic remedies as are usually kept and sold in such stores, but such keeper shall not compound medicines, and medicinal preparations so kept and recognized by the United States Dispensatory shall be compounded by a licensed pharmacist and marked by his label.

SEC. 3127. Any person who shall willfully violate any of the provisions of the preceding sections of this chapter shall forfeit five dollars for each day that he shall continue such violation, one-half to him who shall prosecute to effect and one-half to the town in which the offense was committed.

SEC. 3128. Said commissioners shall have power to examine into all cases of alleged abuse, fraud, and incompetence; cause the prosecution of all persons not complying with the provisions of this chapter, and suspend and revoke the registration of any person legally convicted of violating the same.

SEC. 3129. Every person who shall knowingly adulterate or cause any foreign or inert substance to be mixed with any drug or medicinal substance or preparation recognized by any pharmacopœia, or employed in medicinal or medical practice, so as to weaken or destroy its medicinal effect, or shall sell such drug, compound, or preparation knowing it to be so adulterated or mixed, shall be fined not less than ten nor more than one hundred dollars, and upon conviction all such adulterated or mixed articles in his possession may be seized upon a warrant issued by the court in which such conviction is had, and destroyed by the officer by whom such seizure shall be made.

SEC. 3130. Every person who shall sell arsenic, strychnine, corrosive sublimate, prussic acid, cyanide of potassium shall affix to the package sold by him a label plainly marked with his name, date of sale, and the word "poison," and shall enter on a book kept by him for that purpose the name of the purchaser, date of sale, and the quantity sold; which book shall be kept open for public inspection, carefully preserved; and when he shall close his business or remove from the town in which such business is carried on, or when said book shall be filled with such entries, it shall be deposited by him in the office of the town clerk of the town in which he may conduct his business; and any person who shall violate the preceding provisions of this section, or who when purchasing any of the articles herein named shall give a false or fictitious name to the vender thereof, shall be fined not less than ten nor more than one hundred dollars.

SEC. 3131. Every person who shall sell any of the articles named in the schedule accompanying this section, marked schedule A, except when prescribed by a practising physician, or sold at wholesale to licensed pharmacists, or for use in manufactures or the arts, shall label the bottle, box, or wrapper containing any such article with a label upon which shall be plainly written or printed the word "poison," and any person violating the provisions of this section shall be fined one dollar.

### SCHEDULE A.

Acid carbolic, ammoniated mercury, acid muriatic, chloroform, acid nitric, tinct. aconite, acid sulphuric, tinct. belladonna, acid oxalic, tinct. digitalis, creosote, tinct. opium, extract belladonna, tinct. veratrum viride, sugar of lead, morphine, croton oil, nux vomica, cobalt, extract nux vomica, oil bitter almonds, opium, oil tansy, coculus indicus, aqua ammonia, red oxide mercury, gelsemium, paris green, rat dynamite, rough on rats, or any article like the three last named.

SEC. 3132. Police courts and city courts having criminal jurisdiction where established, and justices of the peace in towns where such courts do not exist, shall hear and determine prosecutions for violations of the provisions of this chapter.

## DISTRICT OF COLUMBIA.

### AN ACT to regulate the practice of pharmacy of the District of Columbia.

*Be it enacted by the Senate and House of Representatives of the United States of America in Congress assembled,* That from and after the passage of this act it shall be unlawful for any person not a registered pharmacist within the meaning of this act, to conduct any pharmacy or store for the purpose of retailing, compounding, or dispensing medicines or poisons, for medical use, in the District of Columbia, except as hereinafter provided.

SECTION 2. That it shall be unlawful for the proprietor of any store or pharmacy to allow any person, except a registered pharmacist, to compound or dispense the prescriptions of physicians, or to retail or dispense poisons for medical use, except as an aid to, and under the immediate supervision of, a registered pharmacist. Any person violating the provisions of this section shall be deemed guilty of a misdemeanor, and, on conviction thereof, shall be liable to a fine of not less than twenty-five dollars nor more than one hundred dollars for each and every such offense.

SEC. 3. That immediately after the passage of this act, and biennially thereafter, or as often as necessary, the Commissioners of the District of Columbia shall appoint three pharmacists and two physicians, all of whom shall have been residents of the District of Columbia for five years, and of at least five years' practical experience in their respective professions, who shall be known and styled as commissioners of pharmacy for the District of Columbia, who shall serve without compensation, and who shall hold office for two years, and until their successors are appointed and qualified. Said commissioners shall, within thirty days after the notification of their appointment, each take and subscribe to an oath to impartially and faithfully discharge their duties as prescribed by this act. The position of any commissioner who shall fail to so qualify within the time named shall be vacant, and the vacancy or vacancies so occurring, or any vacancy or vacancies that may occur, shall be filled by the Commissioners of the District of Columbia.

SEC. 4. That the commissioners of pharmacy shall keep a book of registration open at some convenient place within the city of Washington, of which due notice shall be given through the public press, and shall record therein the name and place of business of every person registered under this act. It shall be the duty of said commissioners of pharmacy to register, without examination, as registered pharmacists all pharmacists and druggists who are engaged in business in the District of Columbia at the passage of this act as owners or principals of stores or pharmacies for selling at retail, compounding, or dispensing drugs, medicines, or chemicals for medicinal use, or for compounding and dispensing physicians' prescriptions, and all assistant pharmacists, twenty-one years of age, engaged in said stores or pharmacies in the District of Columbia at the passage of this act, and who have been engaged as such in some store or pharmacy where physicians' prescriptions were compounded and dispensed for not less than five years prior to the passage of this act: *Provided, however,* That in case of failure or neglect on the part of any such person or persons to present themselves for registration within sixty days after said public notice, they shall undergo an examination such as is provided for in section five of this act.

SEC. 5. That the said commissioners of pharmacy shall, upon application and at such time and place as they may determine, examine each and every person who shall desire to conduct the business of selling at retail, compounding, or dispensing drugs, medicines, or chemicals for medicinal use, or compounding and dispensing physicians' prescriptions within the District of Columbia as pharmacists; and if a majority of said commissioners shall be satisfied that said person is competent and fully qualified to conduct said business of compounding or dispensing drugs, medicines, or chemicals for medicinal use, or to compound and dispense physicians' prescriptions, they shall enter the name of such person as a registered pharmacist in the book provided for in section four of this act.

SEC. 6. That no person shall be entitled to an examination by said commissioners of pharmacy for registration as pharmacist unless he presents satisfactory evidence of being twenty-one years of age and having served not less than four years in a store or pharmacy where physicians' prescriptions were compounded and dispensed, or is a graduate of some respectable medical college or university.

SEC. 7. That all graduates in pharmacy having a diploma from an incorporated college or school of pharmacy that requires a practical experience in pharmacy of not less than four years before granting a diploma, shall be entitled to have their names registered as pharmacists by said commissioners of pharmacy.

SEC. 8. That the commissioners of pharmacy shall be entitled to demand and receive from each person whom they register as pharmacists, without examination, the sum of three dollars, and from each person whom they examine the sum of ten dollars. And in case the examination of said person should prove defective and unsatisfactory, and his name not be registered, he shall be permitted to present himself for reëxamination within any period not exceeding twelve months next thereafter, and no charge shall be made for such reëxamination. The money received under the provisions of this section shall be applied to payment of such expenses as the commissioners may incur in executing the provisions of this act.

SEC. 9. Every registered pharmacist shall be held responsible for the quality of all drugs, chemicals, and medicines he may sell or dispense, with the exception of those sold in the original packages of the manufacturer, and also those known as "patent medicines;" and should he knowingly, intentionally, and fraudulently adulterate, or cause to be adulterated, such drugs, chemicals, or medical preparations, he shall be deemed guilty of a misdemeanor, and, upon conviction thereof, be liable to a penalty not exceeding one hundred dollars, and, in addition thereto, his name shall be stricken from the register.

SEC. 10. It shall be unlawful for any person, from and after the passage of this act, to retail any poisons enumerated in schedules A and B, as follows, to wit:

### SCHEDULE A.

Arsenic and its preparations, corrosive sublimate, white precipitate, red precipitate, biniodide of mercury, cyanide of potassium, hydrocyanic acid, strychnia, and all other poisonous vegetable alkaloids and their salts, essential oil of bitter almonds, opium and its preparations, except paregoric and other preparations of opium containing less than two grains to the ounce.

## SCHEDULE B.

Aconite, belladona, colchicum, conium, nux vomica, henbane, savin, ergot cotton-root, cantharides, creosote, digitalis, and their pharmaceutical preparations, croton-oil, chloroform, chloral hydrate, sulphate of zinc, mineral acids, carbolic acid, and oxalic acid, without distinctly labeling the box, vessel, or paper in which the said poison is contained, and also the outside wrapper or cover, with the name of the article, the word "poison," and the name and place of business of the seller. Nor shall it be lawful for any person to sell or deliver any poisons enumerated in schedules A and B, unless, upon due inquiry, it be found that the purchaser is aware of its poisonous character, and represents that it is to be used for a legitimate purpose. Nor shall it be lawful for any registered pharmacist to sell any poisons included in schedule A without, before delivering the same to the purchaser, causing an entry to be made, in a book kept for that purpose, stating the date of sale, the name and address of the purchaser, the name and quality of the poison sold, the purpose for which it is represented by the purchaser to be required, and the name of the dispenser; such book to be always open for inspection by the proper authorities, and to be preserved for reference for at least five years. The provisions of this section shall not apply to the dispensing of poisons, in not unusual quantities or doses, upon the prescriptions of practitioners of medicine. Nor shall it be lawful for any licensed or registered druggist or pharmacist in the District of Columbia to retail or sell or give away any alcoholic liquors or compounds as a beverage, to be drunk or consumed upon the premises. And any violation of the provisions of this section shall make the owner or principal of said store or pharmacy liable to a fine of not less than twenty-five and not more than one hundred dollars, to be collected in the usual manner.

SEC. 11. Any itinerant vender of any drug, nostrum, ointment, or appliance of any kind, intended for the treatment of diseases or injury, or who shall by writing, or printing, or any other method, publicly professed to cure or treat diseases, injury or deformity, by any drug, nostrum, manipulation, or other expedient, shall pay a license of two hundred dollars per annum into the treasury of the District of Columbia, to be collected in the usual way.

SEC. 12. That any person who shall procure or attempt to procure registration for himself or for another under this act, by making or causing to be made any false representation, shall be deemed guilty of a misdemeanor, and shall, upon conviction thereof, be liable to a penalty of not less than twenty-five nor more than one hundred dollars, and the name of the person so fraudulently registered shall be stricken from the register. Any person not a registered pharmacist as provided for in this act, who shall conduct a store, pharmacy, or place for retailing, compounding or dispensing drugs, medicines, or chemicals for medicinal use, or for compounding, or dispensing physicians' prescriptions, shall be deemed guilty of a misdemeanor, and, upon conviction thereof, shall be liable to a penalty of not less than fifty dollars.

SEC. 13. That all fines and penalties under this act shall be collected in the same manner that other fines and penalties are collected in the District of Columbia; and it shall be the duty of the United States district attorney for the District of Columbia to prosecute all violations of this act.

SEC. 14. That all acts and parts of acts inconsistent with this act be, and the same are hereby, repealed.

Approved June 15, 1878.

## DELAWARE.

### Volume 18, Chapter 36.

AN ACT to regulate the practice of pharmacy in the State of Delaware, and for other purposes.

Whereas the ability of the physicians to overcome disease depends largely upon the obtaining of reliable medicines, intelligently and skillfully prepared; and

Whereas, from time to time, unskilled and incompetent persons engage in the compounding and sale of drugs, medicines, and chemicals to the endangering of the health and lives of the public.

*Be it enacted by the Senate and House of Representatives of the State of Delaware in General Assembly met:*

SECTION 1. That from and after the passage of this act it shall be unlawful for any person to open, conduct, or manage within the corporate limits of any town in this State any pharmacy, drug store, or other place for the retailing, compounding, or dispensing of drugs, medicines, or poisons, unless such person shall be registered as a pharmacist under the provisions of this act. Nor shall the sale of patent, quack, or proprietary articles be lawful, except in regular licensed stores under a penalty of ten dollars for each and every offense.

SEC. 2. In order to become registered as a proprietor or manager of a pharmacy the applicant must be a graduate of a college of pharmacy or medicine of good standing. Otherwise he shall have had three years' continuous practical experience in the retail drug business, and shall submit to, and satisfactorily pass, an examination before the State board of pharmacy.

SEC. 3. No person who shall conduct or manage any pharmacy, drug store, or other place for the retailing, compounding, or dispensing of drugs, medicines, or poisons for medical use shall permit or suffer at any time any clerk or other employé to be left in charge of same unless said person be a registered assistant, with one year's continuous practical experience or an examination certificate from the board of pharmacy. Nor shall any proprietor or manager of any pharmacy permit any clerk or other person who has had less than one year's practical experience in the retail drug business to compound or dispense any physician's prescriptions, except under the immediate directions of the proprietor or manager. Any person who shall not comply with the provisions of this section shall be deemed guilty of a misdemeanor, and, upon conviction thereof, shall be fined not less than twenty dollars nor more than fifty dollars for each day whereon such violation occurs or is continued, one-half of fine imposed to go to the State board of pharmacy and the balance to the county in which such violation occurs.

SEC. 4. Every dispenser of drugs shall keep a record of all sales of strychnia, arsenic, and corrosive sublimate, said record to be open to proper legal inspection. Any person failing to comply with the provisions of this section shall be deemed guilty of a misdemeanor, and, upon conviction thereof, shall be fined five dollars for each and every offense.

SEC. 5. The Pharmaceutical Society of Delaware shall on or before the first day of June, eighteen hundred and eighty-seven, recommend to the governor the names of at least six graduates of a college of pharmacy of good standing and four graduates of medicine, and it shall be the duty of the governor on or before the day and year aforesaid to appoint, in writing, three of the former and two of the latter to constitute the State board of pharmacy. The said board shall have authority to act from and after the first day of July aforesaid. The members so appointed shall hold their offices for five years: *Provided,* That the term of office for the first five appointed shall be so arranged that the time of one shall expire on the first day of July of each year, and the vacancies so created, as well as all vacancies occurring, shall, with or without recommendation aforesaid, be filled by appointment by the governor of a person or persons possessing the like qualifications as his or their predecessors in office. The person or persons so appointed to hold office during the remainder of the term for which his or their predecessor or predecessors were appointed. Before entering upon the discharge of their official duties the members of said board shall be duly sworn or affirmed for the faithful and impartial performance of their duties as such members. Any three members shall constitute a quorum for the transaction of business. The said board shall meet at least once in every three months, and it shall be its duty to examine into the qualifications of all applicants and register them accordingly, keeping correct record of all official transactions, and to report annually to the governor prior to the first day of July of each year.

SEC. 6. The members of said board shall receive no compensation, but may pay the expenses incurred by them in the discharge of official duty out of any money coming to said board under the provisions of this act. The said board before issuing a certificate of registration to any pharmacist or assistant shall, if the applicant be entitled to be registered without the passage of an examination, receive from such applicant the sum of one dollar; but if the applicant be required, under the provisions of this act, to pass an examination he shall pay to said board the sum of five dollars.

SEC. 7. Any person not being a registered pharmacist, or having in his employ one who is not registered according to the meaning of this act, who shall, thirty days after this act takes effect, keep a pharmacy or store for compounding or retailing drugs or medicines, shall be deemed guilty of a misdemeanor, and upon conviction thereof shall be fined the sum of fifty dollars.

SEC. 8. Any person who shall violate any of the provisions of this act shall be deemed guilty of a misdemeanor, and upon conviction thereof in the court of general sessions of the peace and jail delivery shall be fined, according to the amount specified after the section violated, for each day whereon such violation occurs or is continued. One-half of the fine imposed to go to the State board of pharmacy and the balance to the county in which such violation occurs.

SEC. 9. Nothing in this act contained shall be taken to render unlawful the compounding by any physician of prescriptions to be used by him in his own practice.

SEC. 10. That an act entitled "An act to regulate the practice of pharmacy in the State of Delaware," passed at Dover, April 17, 1883, be and the same is hereby repealed: *Provided, however,* That nothing in this act contained shall prevent the registration of those pharmacists now already engaged in the drug business in towns not affected by repealed act. Nor shall in any manner affect the right of any person to whom a certificate of registration has heretofore been duly issued under said repealed act: *And provided further,* That the State board of pharmacy, organized under the repealed act, shall continue to exist in the same manner and with the same power as shall be possessed by board provided by this act until July first, eighteen hundred and eighty-seven, any vacancy or vacancies now existing, or hereafter occurring, during existence of old board shall be filled by appointment by the governor of a person possessing like qualifications of his predecessor, who shall also be qualified by oath; also that all money, records, and effects belonging to old board shall be turned over to their successors.

SEC. 11. *Provided, also,* That nothing in this act shall prohibit the sale of standard proprietary medicines by general stores.

Passed at Dover, April 14, 1887.

## VOLUME XIX, CHAPTER 123.

AN ACT to amend chapter 36, volume 18, Laws of Delaware, entitled "An act to regulate the practice of pharmacy in the State of Delaware, and for other purposes," and to further amend chapter 549, volume 18, Laws of Delaware, entitled "An act to amend certain portions of the laws governing the practice of pharmacy in the State of Delaware."

*Be it enacted by the Senate and House of Representatives of the State of Delaware in General Assembly met:*

SECTION 1. Amend section 3, chapter 36, volume 18, Laws of Delaware, by striking out of said section the words "A registered assistant with one year continuous practical experience, or an examination certificate from the board of pharmacy," beginning in line six and ending in line eight, and inserting in lieu thereof the following: "Registered as a proprietor or manager according to the provisions of section 2, chapter 36, volume 18, Laws of Delaware, or be registered as a qualified assistant according to the provisions hereinafter stated."

In order to become registered as a qualified assistant the applicant shall have had three years' continuous practical experience in the retail drug business, or shall submit to and satisfactorily pass an examination before the State board of pharmacy; also, amend section 5 of said act by striking out in line 1 the words, "The Pharmaceutical Society of Delaware," and inserting in lieu thereof the following: "The Delaware Pharmaceutical Society."

SEC. 2. Further amend section 1, chapter 549, volume 18, Laws of Delaware, by striking out all portions of said section conflicting with section 1 of this act.

SEC. 3. *Provided*, That nothing in this act contained shall prevent any person already registered as assistant under previous acts from enjoying all the privileges granted by said previous acts at the time of such registration.

Passed at Dover, April 28, 1891.

## VOLUME 18, CHAPTER 549.

AN ACT to amend certain portions of the laws governing the practice of pharmacy in the State of Delaware.

*Be it enacted by the Senate and House of Representatives of the State of Delaware in General Assembly met:*

SECTION 1. Amend section 3 of chapter 36, volume 18, Laws of Delaware, by striking out the word "one" where the same occurs in lines 6 and 10 of the said section and by inserting in lieu thereof the word "two."

SEC. 2. Further amend the said act by striking out all of section 5 after the word "years" in line 11 and before the word "the" in line 17 of said section and by inserting in lieu thereof the following: "*Provided*, That the term of office for the first five appointed shall be arranged by lot, so that the time of one shall expire on the first day of July of each year, and the vacancies so created, as well as all vacancies occurring, shall, with recommendation aforesaid, be filled by appointment by the governor of a person or persons possessing like qualifications as his or their predecessor in office.

Passed at Dover, April 25, 1889.

## FLORIDA.

### PHARMACY LAW.

AN ACT to regulate the practice of pharmacy in cities and towns of more than two hundred inhabitants, and the sale of poisons in the State of Florida, and to affix penalties.

*Be it enacted by the Legislature of the State of Florida:*

SECTION 1. That from and after the passage of this act it shall be unlawful for any person, not a registered pharmacist, within the meaning of this act, to conduct any pharmacy, drug store, apothecary shop or store located in any village, town, or city in the State of Florida of more than two hundred inhabitants, or within two miles of any incorporated city or town of more than two hundred inhabitants, for the purpose of retailing, compounding, or dispensing medicines or poisons for medical use, except as hereinafter provided.

SEC. 2. *Be it further enacted*, That it shall be unlawful for the proprietor of any store or pharmacy in any village, town, or city in the State of Florida of more than two hundred inhabitants, or within two miles of any incorporated city or town of more than two hundred inhabitants, to allow any person except a registered pharmacist to compound or dispense the prescriptions of physicians, or to retail or dispense poisons for medical use except as an aid to and under the supervision of a registered pharmacist. Any person violating the provisions of this section shall be deemed guilty of a misdemeanor, and on conviction shall be liable to a fine of not less than $25 nor more than $100 for each and every offense.

SEC. 3. *Be it further enacted,* That the governor shall appoint five persons from among the most prominent pharmacists of the State, all of whom shall have been residents of the State for two years, and of at least five years' practical experience in their profession, who shall be known and styled "Board of pharmacy State of Florida," one of whom shall hold his office for one year, one for two years, one for three years, two for four years, each, until his successor shall be appointed and qualified; and each year thereafter another commissioner shall be so appointed for four years and until a successor is appointed and qualified. If a vacancy occurs in said board, another commissioner shall be appointed, as aforesaid, to fill the unexpired term thereof. Said board shall have power to make by-laws and all necessary regulations, and to create auxiliary boards if necessary, for the proper fulfillment of their duties under this act without expense to the State.

SEC. 4. *Be it further enacted,* That the board of pharmacy shall register in a suitable book the names and places of residences of all persons to whom they issue certificates, and dates thereof. It shall be the duty of said board of pharmacy to register without examination, as registered pharmacists, all pharmacists and druggists who are engaged in business in the State of Florida, at the passage of this act, as owners or principals of stores or pharmacies in any village, town, or city of more than two hundred inhabitants, for selling at retail, compounding or dispensing drugs, medicines, or chemicals for medical use, or compounding or dispensing physicians' prescriptions, and all assistant pharmacists over eighteen years of age, engaged in said stores or pharmacies in any village, town, or city of more than two hundred inhabitants in the State of Florida, at the passage of this act, and have been engaged two years as such in some store or pharmacy where physicians' prescriptions were compounded or dispensed: *Provided, however,* That in case of failure or neglect on the part of any person or persons to apply for registration within sixty days after they shall have been notified by said board of pharmacy for the State of Florida, they shall undergo an examination as is provided for in section 5 of this act.

SEC. 5. *Be it further enacted,* That the said board of pharmacy shall, upon application of ten applicants for examination, and at such time and place and in such manner as they may determine, either by a schedule of questions to be answered and subscribed to under oath, or orally, examine each and every person who shall desire to conduct the business of selling at retail, compounding or dispensing drugs, medicines, or chemicals for medical use, or for compounding or dispensing physicians' prescriptions as pharmacists, and if a majority of said board shall be satisfied that such person is competent and fully qualified to conduct said business of compounding or dispensing drugs, medicines, or chemicals for medical use, or to compound or dispense physicians' prescriptions, they shall enter the name of such person as a registered pharmacist in a book provided for in section 4 of this act; and that all graduates of colleges of pharmacy that require a practical experience in pharmacy of not less than four years before granting a diploma, shall be entitled to have their names registered by said board without examination: *Provided, however,* That this act shall not be so construed as to prevent any physician who is authorized to practice medicine or surgery under the laws of this State from registering as a pharmacist or druggist without examination: *Provided,* That any person or persons not a pharmacist or druggist may open and conduct such store if he or they keep constantly in their employ a registered pharmacist or druggist; but shall not himself or themselves sell or dispense drugs or medicine, except proprietary patent medicines in original packages.

SEC. 6. *Be it further enacted,* That the board of pharmacy shall be entitled to demand and receive of each person whom they register and furnish a certificate as a registered pharmacist, without examination, the sum of two dollars, and for each and every person that they examine orally, on whose answers to a schedule of questions are returned, subscribed under oath, the sum of three dollars, which shall be in full for services; and in case the examination of said person shall prove defective and unsatisfactory, and his name not be registered, he shall be permitted to present himself for examination within any period not exceeding twelve months thereafter, and no charge shall be made for such examination.

SEC. 7. *Be it further enacted,* That every registered pharmacist, apothecary, and owner of any store shall be held responsible for the quality of all drugs, chemicals, or medicines he may sell or dispense, with the exception of those sold in original packages of the manufacturer, and also those known as proprietary, and should he knowingly intermingle and fraudulently adulterate, or cause to be adulterated, such drugs, chemicals, or medical preparations, he shall be deemed guilty of a misdemeanor, and upon conviction thereof be liable to a penalty not exceeding $100, and, in addition thereto, his name shall be stricken from the register.

SEC. 8. *Be it further enacted,* That it shall be unlawful for any person not a registered pharmacist, from and after sixty days after the passage of this act, to retail any poisons enumerated below: Arsenic and its preparations, corrosive sublimate, white and red precipitate, biniodide of mercury, cyannide of potassium, hydrocyanic acid, strychnine, and all other poisonous vegetable alkaloids, and their salts, and the essential oil of almonds, opium and its preparations, except paregoric and other preparations of opium containing less than two grains to the ounce; aconite, belladonna, colchium, conium, nux vomica, henbane, savin, ergot, cotton root, cantharides, creosote, veratrum digitalis, and their pharmaceutical preparations; croton oil, chloroform, chloral hydrate, sulphate of zinc, mineral acids, carbolic and oxalic acids; and he shall label the box, vessel, or paper in which said poison is contained with the name of the article, the word "poison," and the name and place of business of the seller. Nor shall it be lawful for any persons to deliver or sell any poisons enumerated above, unless upon due inquiry it be found that the purchaser is aware of its poisonous character and represents that it is to be used for a legitimate purpose. The provisions of this section shall not apply to the dispensing of poisons in not unusual quantities or doses upon the prescription of practitioners of medicine. Any violation of this section shall make the principal of said store liable to a fine of not less than $10 or more than $100: *Provided, however,* That this section shall not apply to manufacturers making and selling at wholesale any of the above poisons: *And provided,* That each box, vessel, or paper in which said poison is contained shall be labeled with the name of the article, the word "poison," and the name and place of business of the seller.

SEC. 9. *Be it further enacted,* That any itinerant vendor of any drug, poison, ointment, or appliance of any kind intended for treatment of any disease, or injury or deformity, by any drug, nostrum, or manipulation or other expedient, shall pay a license of $500 per annum to the State, to be paid in the manner for obtaining public license according to the usual laws in force for that purpose.

SEC. 10. *Be it further enacted,* That any person who shall procure, or attempt to procure, registration for himself or for another under this act by making, or causing to be made, false representations, shall be guilty of a misdemeanor, and shall, upon conviction thereof, be liable to a penalty of not less than $25 nor more than $100, and the name of the person so falsely registered shall be stricken from the register. Any person not a registered pharmacist, as provided for in this act, who shall conduct such a store, pharmacy, or other place for retailing, compounding, or dispensing drugs, medicines, or chemicals for medical use, or for compounding or dispensing physicians' prescriptions, or who shall take, use, or exhibit the title of registered pharmacist, shall be guilty of a misdemeanor, and upon conviction thereof shall be liable to a penalty of not less than $100.

SEC. 11. This act shall not apply to physicians putting up their own prescriptions.

SEC. 12. *Be it further enacted,* That it shall be the duty of every registered pharmacist to conspicuously post his certificate of registration in his place of business.

Any person who shall fail to comply with all the provisions of this section shall be liable to a fine of $5 for each calendar month during which he is delinquent.

SEC. 13. The sum of $500 per year, or as much thereof as may be found necessary, is hereby appropriated out of the money so received for license for the expense of said board of pharmacy. All surplus over and above said amount to be divided as follows: One-half to the "Florida State Pharmaceutical Association," the remainder to be paid into the State treasury.

SEC. 14. All suits for the recovery of the several penalties prescribed in this act shall be presented in the name of the State of Florida in any court having jurisdiction, and it shall be the duty of the State's attorney of the county wherein such offense is committed to present all persons violating the provisions of this act upon proper complaint being made.

SEC. 15. *Be it further enacted,* That all laws and parts of laws in conflict with the provisions of this act be, and the same are hereby, repealed.

Approved May 30, 1889.

## FLORIDA DRUG LAW.

2668. Adulterations of drugs.—Whoever fraudulently adulterates for the purpose of sale, any drug or medicine, or sells any fraudulently adulterated drug or medicine, knowing the same to be adulterated, shall be punished by imprisonment not exceeding one year, or by fine not exceeding four hundred dollars; and such adulterated drugs and medicines shall be forfeited and destroyed under the direction of the court, and if the offender be a registered pharmacist his name shall be stricken from the register.

## GEORGIA.

AN ACT to establish the Georgia State board of pharmacy, and to prescribe the powers and duties of said board, and to regulate the compounding and vending of medicines, drugs, and poisons in the State of Georgia, and to provide a penalty for the infringement of the provisions of this act.

SECTION 1. *The General Assembly of the State of Georgia do enact,* That, within sixty days after the passage of this act, the governor of the State shall appoint five experienced druggists or practical pharmacists, from the names of ten persons suggested by the Georgia pharmaceutical association, who shall have been actively engaged in the drug business within this State for the last three years immediately preceding their appointment, and these five druggists or practical pharmacists, so appointed, shall constitute the Georgia State board of pharmacy, one of whom shall hold his office for one year, one for two years, one for three years, one for four years, and one for five years, until his successor shall have been appointed and qualified. And at each and every annual meeting thereafter the said Georgia pharmaceutical association shall submit to the governor the names of five persons with the qualifications hereinbefore mentioned, and the governor shall appoint, from the names so submitted, one member of said board, who shall hold his office for five years, until his successor is appointed and qualified. (This amendment not to affect the term of office of the present board.)

SEC. 2. *Be it further enacted,* That immediately, and before entering upon the duties of said office, the members of said board shall take the oath prescribed by the constitution of the State for State officers, and shall file the same in the office of the secretary of State, who, upon receiving the said oaths of office, shall issue to each of said examiners a certificate of appointment.

SEC. 3. *Be it further enacted,* That immediately after the appointment and qualification of said board, they shall meet and organize as a State board of pharmacy, elect a chairman and secretary, and adopt such rules, regulations, and by-laws as they shall deem necessary to carry into execution the provisions of this act.

SEC. 4. *Be it further enacted,* That said board shall meet at least once every twelve months at such place as a majority of the board may determine, and that the board may also hold special meetings as frequently, and at such places, as the proper discharge of the duties shall require; the same to be convened by order of the chairman, and the rules or by-laws shall provide for the giving of proper notice of the time and place of all such meetings to the members of the board and to the board.

Sec. 5. "It shall be the duty of the Georgia State board of pharmacy to grant license: First, to druggists who, after three years' experience in a drug store managed by a licensed apothecary or pharmacist, shall have passed a satisfactory examination before the said board of pharmacy. Second, to such physicians, graduates of a regular medical college, and such graduates of schools of pharmacy as shall have passed a satisfactory examination before said board of pharmacy. Third, to pharmacists who have obtained license from such other State boards of pharmacy as may be recognized by said Georgia State board of pharmacy. All licenses granted shall be signed by a majority of the whole board; shall specify the ground upon which said license is granted; shall be in such form as the board shall prescribe, and shall be posted in a conspicuous place in the place of business of such licentiate: *Provided*, That this act shall not apply to physicians who are graduates of medical colleges in good standing, and who have been practicing medicine for five years at the time of the passage of this act." *

Sec. 6. *Be it further enacted*, That all persons applying for examination and license shall pay to the board of pharmacy the sum of five dollars, and if passing the examination, shall be furnished with the license as hereinbefore provided, and an annual renewal fee of two dollars shall be paid to keep the same in force. Should the applicant fail to stand a satisfactory examination no fee shall be required for a subsequent examination, such subsequent examination not to be granted within six months after the first. And it shall be the duty of the board to keep a record of its transactions in a book to be kept for that purpose by the secretary, said book to be turned over to their successors in office. All moneys received by said board from renewal fees, in excess of six hundred dollars, shall be paid to the treasurer of the Georgia pharmaceutical association. Said board shall make an annual report to the Georgia pharmaceutical association.

Sec. 7. *Be it further enacted*, That all persons now lawfully engaged in the compounding and vending of medicines, drugs, and poisons in this State, shall, on or before December 1st, 1881, and every person who shall be hereafter duly licensed under the provisions of this act, shall, before engaging in any business under said license, register in the office of the ordinary of the county wherein he resides or intends to conduct said business, in a book to be kept for that purpose by said ordinary, his name, nationality, and credentials, and date thereof, under which he is entitled to engage in such vocation. For each registration the ordinary shall receive fifty cents, to be paid by the party so registering, and a certificate of such registration, stating the terms of same, shall be given him by said ordinary.

Sec. 8. *Be it further enacted*, That no person shall engage in the compounding or vending of medicines, drugs, or poisons within this State without a full compliance with this act, except (1) such druggists as are exempt from the operations of the present law by the statutes of the State of Georgia, and such druggists as have heretofore obtained license, and are legally authorized by existing laws to compound and vend drugs, poisons, and chemicals; (2) physicians putting up their own prescriptions, and dispensing medicines from their own office; (3) merchants selling

---

*THE EFFECT OF THIS SECTION.

Under this amendment, the board can not grant licenses on diplomas (either M. D. or PH. G.) as formerly, except to those physicians who had been practicing five years at the passage of this act. In other words, only physicians who graduated prior to 1887 and can prove continuous practice for five years are entitled to registration without examination; others must pass the examination to register as druggists.

Approved October 20, 1891.

family medicines not poison, as prescribed and allowed by section 1409 of the code of 1873 of Georgia; (4) assistants in drug stores where the manager has complied with the requirements of this act.

SEC. 9. No person shall within this State manufacture for sale, offer for sale, or sell any drug, medicine, chemical, or pharmaceutical preparation which is adulterated. A drug, medicine, chemical, or pharmaceutical preparation shall be deemed to be adulterated: (1) If, when sold under or by a name recognized in the U. S. Pharmacopœia, it differs from the standard in strength, quality, or purity laid down therein; (2) if, when sold under or by a name not recognized in the U. S. Pharmacopœia, but which is found in some other standard work, it differs materially from the standard of strength, quality, or purity laid down in such work; (3) if its strength, quality, or purity falls below the professed standard.

SEC. 10. Every person manufacturing, offering for sale, or selling any drug, medicine, or pharmaceutical preparation shall furnish to the State board of pharmacy, or any person interested or demanding the same, who shall tender him the value of the same, a sample sufficient for the analysis of any such drug, medicine, chemical, or pharmaceutical preparation which is in his possession.

SEC. 11. On complaint being made, the board of pharmacy is hereby empowered to employ an export chemist or analyst to examine into the so-claimed adulteration and report upon the result of his investigation, and if said report justify such action the board shall cause the prosecution of the offender; and any person found guilty of adulteration as defined by this act shall be adjudged to pay, in addition to the fine hereinafter provided for, all necessary costs and expense incurred in inspecting and analyzing such adulterated articles which said person may have been found guilty of manufacturing, selling, or offering for sale, and it shall be the duty of the solicitor to prosecute all violations of this act.

SEC. 12. *Be it further enacted,* That any person who shall violate the provisions of this act, or shall register fraudulently, shall be guilty of a misdemeanor, and upon conviction shall be punished by a fine not to exceed one hundred dollars, imprisonment not to exceed three months, either or both, at the discretion of the court. In all cases of prosecution under this act the burden shall be upon the defendant to show his authority.

SEC. 13. *Be it further enacted,* That all fees for examination and license, and one-half of the fines collected from convictions under this act, shall be paid to the State board of pharmacy, to defray the expenses of the same, and as compensation for their services.

SEC. 14. *Be it further enacted,* That this act shall take effect from and after the date of its passage.

SEC. 15. Repeals conflicting laws.

Approved September 28, 1881.

ALFRED H. COLQUITT,
*Governor.*

Sections 1, 3, 5, 6, and 12 amended, and sections 9, 10, and 11 added.
Approved October 25, 1889.

JOHN B. GORDON,
*Governor.*

## ILLEGAL SALE OF OPIUM.

AN ACT to prevent the sale of opium and its preparations to persons habitually addicted to its use.

SECTION 1. *Be it enacted by the General Assembly of the State of Georgia,* That it shall not be lawful for any druggist, pharmacist, or other person selling opium and its preparations by retail, to sell, give, or furnish directly, or indirectly, opium, or its preparations, containing more than two grains of opium to the ounce, in any quantity, to any person addicted to its use, after a written notice from a near relative of such person that he or she is habitually addicted to its use, except upon the written prescription of a physician setting forth the necessity of its purchase, and showing the good faith of the prescription.

SEC. 2. *Be it further enacted by the authority aforesaid,* That any person violating the provisions of this section shall be guilty of a misdemeanor, and upon conviction shall be punished as prescribed in section 4310 of the code

SEC. 3. *Be it further enacted by the authority aforesaid,* That all laws and parts of laws in conflict with this act be, and the same are hereby, repealed.

Approved September 6, 1887.

## AN ACT to regulate the sale of poisons in this State.

SECTION 1. *Be it enacted by the General Assembly of the State of Georgia,* That from and after the first day of May, 1876, it shall be unlawful for any person to furnish by retail any poison enumerated in the schedules "A" and "B," as follows, to wit:

Schedule "A"—Arsenic and its preparations—corrosive sublimate, white precipitate, red precipitate, biniodide of mercury, cyanide of potassium, hydrocyanic acid, strychnia, and all other poisonous vegetable alkaloids and their salts; essential oil of bitter almonds; opium and its preparation, except paregoric and other preparations of opium containing less than two grains to the ounce.

Schedule "B"—Aconite, belladonna, colchicum, conium, nux vomica, henbane, savin, ergot, cotton root, cantharides, creosote, digitalis, and their pharmaceutical preparations, croton oil, chloroform, chloral hydrate, sulphate of zinc, mineral acids, carbolic acid, and oxalic acid, without distinctly labeling the bottle, box, vessel, or paper in which said poison is contained, and also the outside wrapper or cover thereof with the name of the article, the word "poison," and the name and place of business of him or her who furnishes the same; nor unless, upon due inquiry, it be found that the person to whom it is delivered is aware of its poisonous character, and represents that it is to be used for a legitimate purpose.

SEC. 2. *Be it further enacted by the authority aforesaid,* That no licensed or registered druggist or pharmacist shall, after said date, sell or deliver any of the poisons included in the schedule "A" without, before delivering the same, causing an entry to be made in a book kept for that purpose, stating the date of delivery, the name and address of the person receiving the same, the name and quantity of the poison, the purpose for which it is represented by each person to be required, and the name of the dispenser. Such book shall be always open for inspection by the proper authorities, and be preserved for reference for at least five years.

SEC. 3. *Be it further enacted by the authority aforesaid,* That nothing in this act shall apply to the dispensing of poison in not unusual quantities or doses, upon the prescriptions of practitioners of medicine.

SEC. 4. *Be it further enacted by the authority aforesaid,* That any person violating the provisions of this act shall be guilty of a misdemeanor, and upon conviction thereof, in any court in this State, shall be punished by fine not exceeding one thousand dollars, or imprisonment not exceeding six months in jail, or both, in the discretion of the judge pronouncing the sentence.

SEC. 5. Repeals conflicting laws.

### SCHEDULE A.

ARSENIC—
    Fowler's solution.
    Donovan's solution.
    Arsenious acid.
    Arsenite ammonia.
    Tinct. opii deodorata.
    Tinct. opii acetata.
    Vine of.
    Wine of.
    Fluid and solid extract of.
ACID, PRUSSIC—
    Potassium cyanide.

MERCURY BINIODIDE—
    Corrosive sublimate.
    Red precipitate.
    White precipitate.
STRYCHNINE—
    Sulphate.
    Muriate.
MORPHIA—
    Acetate.
    Bromide.
    Muriate.
    Sulphate.

SCHEDULE A—continued.

MORPHIA—Continued.
    Valerianate,
      and other solutions.
    Oil bitter almonds.
OPIUM—
    Laudanum.
ALKALOIDS—
    Aconitia.

Atropia.
Brucia.
Codeia.
Conia.
Emetia.
Narcotina.
Nicotia.
Veratria, etc.

## SCHEDULE B.

ACONITE—
    Belladonna.
    Cantharides.
    Colchicum root.
    Colchicum seed.
    Cotton root.
    Digitalis.
    Ergot.
    Henbane.
    Nux vomica.
    Savin,
      including their—
    Tinctures, fluid and
    Solid extracts,
    Wines and oils.

Carbolic acid and solution.
Chloral hydrate.
Chloroform.
Creosote.
Croton oil.
Chromic acid.
Muriatic acid.
Nitric acid.
Nitrous acid.
Nitro-muriatic acid.
Oxalic acid.
Phosphoric acid.
Sulphuric acid.
Sulphurous acid.
Sulphate zinc.

## LAW REGULATING THE SALE OF MORPHINE.—NO. 384.

AN ACT to prescribe the manner of selling the sulphate and other preparations of morphine in this State, and for other purposes.

SECTION 1. *Be it enacted by the General Assembly of the State of Georgia*, That on and after the first day of January, 1886, it shall not be lawful for any druggist or other dealer in drugs and medicines to sell or offer for sale any sulphate or other preparations of morphine in any bottle, vial, envelope, or other package, unless the same be wrapped in a scarlet paper or envelope, and all bottles or vials used for the above purpose shall have, in addition to said scarlet paper wrapper, a scarlet label lettered in white letters, plainly naming the contents of said bottle.

SEC. 2. *Be it further enacted by the authority aforesaid,* That any one violating the provisions of the above section shall be guilty of a misdemeanor, and on conviction thereof shall be fined not less than ten nor more than fifty dollars, at the discretion of the court, for each and every violation of the preceding section.

SEC. 3. *Be it further enacted,* That all laws or part of laws in conflict with this act be, and the same are hereby, repealed.

Approved, October 15, 1885.

### SECTION 3004 OF THE CODE.

Adulterated drugs.—"A person who knowingly or carelessly, by himself or his agents, sells to another adulterated drugs or liquors by the use of which damage accrues to the purchaser, or his patients, or his family, or his property, shall be liable in damages for the injury done."

# IDAHO.

Has no pharmacy law.

# ILLINOIS.

**AN ACT to regulate the practice of pharmacy in the State of Illinois.**

SECTION 1. *Be it enacted by the people of the State of Illinois, represented in the General Assembly,* That it shall not be lawful for any person, other than a registered pharmacist, to retail, compound, or dispense drugs, medicines, or poisons, or to open or conduct any pharmacy or store for retailing, compounding, or dispensing drugs, medicines, or poisons, unless such person shall be, or shall employ and place in charge of said pharmacy or store, a registered pharmacist, within the meaning of this act, except as hereinafter provided.

SEC. 2. Any person shall be entitled to be registered as a registered pharmacist, within the meaning of this act, who shall be a licentiate in pharmacy, or shall furnish satisfactory evidence to the State board of pharmacy that he has had five years' practical experience in compounding drugs in a drug store or pharmacy where the prescriptions of medical practitioners are compounded. The said board shall have the right to refuse registration to applicants whose examination or credentials are not satisfactory evidence of their competency. This provision shall also apply to the registration of assistant pharmacists hereinafter mentioned. (As amended by act approved June 4, 1889; in force July 1, 1889.)

SEC. 3. Graduates in pharmacy must be such persons as have had four years' practical experience in drug stores where the prescriptions of medical practitioners are compounded, and have obtained a satisfactory diploma or credentials of their attainments from a regularly incorporated college or school of pharmacy.

SEC. 4. Licentiates in pharmacy must be persons not less than 18 years of age, who have had three years' practical experience in compounding drugs in drug stores where the prescriptions of medical practitioners are compounded, and have passed a satisfactory examination before the State board of pharmacy hereinafter mentioned. The said board may, in their discretion, grant certificates of registration to such persons as shall furnish, with their application, satisfactory proof that they have been registered by examination in some other State: *Provided,* That such other State shall require a degree of competency equal to that required of applicants in this State. (As amended by act approved June 4, 1889; in force July 1, 1889.)

SEC. 5. The governor, with the advice and consent of the Senate, shall appoint five persons from among such competent pharmacists in the State as have had ten years' practical experience in the dispensing of physicians' prescriptions, who shall constitute the board of pharmacy. The persons so appointed shall hold their offices for five years: *Provided,* That the term of office of the five first appointed shall be so arranged that the term of one shall expire on the thirtieth day of December of each year; and the vacancies so created, as well as all vacancies otherwise occurring, shall be filled by the governor, with the advice and consent of the Senate: *And provided, also,* That appointments made when the Senate is not in session, may be confirmed at its next ensuing session. The Illinois pharmaceutical association shall annually report directly to the governor, recommending the first year the names of at least ten persons, whom said association shall deem best qualified to serve as members of the board of pharmacy, and the names of at least three persons each year thereafter, to fill any vacancies which shall occur in said board.

SEC. 6. The said board shall, within thirty days after its appointment, meet and organize by electing a president from among their members, and a secretary, who shall not be a member of said board. The board shall also elect a treasurer who is a member of the board. Said board shall prescribe the duties and compensation of such treasurer, and shall require the said treasurer to give such bond as the said board shall direct. The secretary shall pay over to the treasurer all moneys that shall come into his hands as such secretary. It shall be the duty of the board to examine all applications for registration submitted in proper form; to grant certificates of registration to such persons as may be entitled to the same under the provisions of this act; to cause the prosecution of all persons violating its provisions; to report annually to the governor and to the Illinois pharmaceutical association upon the condition of pharmacy in this State, which said report shall also furnish a record of the proceedings of the said board for the year, and also the names of all the pharmacists duly registered under this act. The board shall hold meetings for the examination of applicants for registration and the transaction of such other business as shall pertain to its duties, at least once in six months: *Provided*, That said board shall hold meetings once in every year in the city of Chicago, and in the city of Springfield, and it shall give thirty days' public notice of the time and place of such meeting; shall have power to make by-laws for the proper fulfillment of its duties under this act, and shall keep a book of registration, in which shall be entered the names and places of business of all persons registered under this act, which book shall also specify such facts as said persons shall claim to justify their registration. Three members of said board shall constitute a quorum. (As amended by act approved June 4, 1889; in force July 1, 1889.)

SEC. 7. Licentiates in pharmacy shall, at the time of passing their examination, be registered by the Secretary of the State board of pharmacy as registered pharmacists. (As amended by act approved June 4, 1889; in force July 1, 1889.)

SEC. 8. Any person shall be entitled to registration as assistant pharmacist who is of the age of 18 years, of good moral character, temperate habits, and has had three years' service under a registered pharmacist, and the time of attendance at any respectable school of pharmacy shall be accredited on the above time, or shall pass an examination before the State board of pharmacy that shall show competency or qualification equal to such service. Each applicant for registration by examination as assistant pharmacist shall pay to said board the sum of five dollars before receiving his certificate of registration. Applicants other than by examination shall pay to the board a fee of one dollar. Any assistant pharmacist shall have the right to act as clerk or salesman in a drug store or pharmacy during the temporary absence of the owner or manager thereof. (As amended by act approved June 4, 1889; in force July 1, 1889.)

SEC. 9. Every person applying for the registration of a registered pharmacist, shall, before a certificate is granted, pay to the secretary of the board the sum of two dollars; and a like sum shall be paid by licentiates of other boards who shall apply for registration; and by every applicant for registration by examination shall be paid the sum of five dollars: *Provided*, That in case of the failure of any applicant to pass a satisfactory examination, his money shall be refunded. (As amended by act approved June 4, 1889; in force July 1, 1889.)

SEC. 10. Every registerd pharmacist who desires to continue the practice of his profession, shall annually thereafter during the time he shall continue in such practice, on such date as the board of pharmacy may determine, of which date he shall have thirty days' notice by said board, pay to the secretary of the board a registration fee, to be fixed by the board, but which shall in no case exceed $1.00, for which he shall receive a renewal of said registration. The failure of any registered pharmacist to pay said fee shall not deprive him of his right to renewal upon payment thereof; nor shall his retirement from the profession deprive him of the right to renew his registration should he at any time thereafter wish to resume the practice, upon the payment of said fee. Registered assistants, upon receiving notice as aforesaid, shall, if they desire to renew their registration, pay to the secretary of said board an annual fee of one dollar. Every certificate of registration granted under this act shall be conspicuously exposed in the pharmacy to which it applies. (As amended by act approved June 4, 1889; in force July 1, 1889.)

SEC. 11. The secretary of the board shall receive a salary which shall be fixed by the board, and which shall not exceed the sum of fifteen hundred dollars (1,500) per year; he shall also receive his traveling and other expenses incurred in the performance of his official duties. The members of the board shall receive the sum of $5 for each day actually engaged in this service and all legitimate and necessary expenses incurred in attending the meetings of said board. Said expenses shall be paid from the fees and penalties received by the board, under the provisions of this act, and no part of the salary or other expenses of the board shall be paid out of the State treasury. All moneys received in excess of said per diem allowance and other expenses above provided for shall be held by the treasurer as a special fund for meeting the expenses of said board, and the cost of an annual report of the proceedings of the Illinois pharmaceutical association, and the necessary expenses of said association: *Provided*, That when the amount of money in the hands of the treasurer at any time exceeds two thousand dollars, the amount of such excess shall be paid into the State treasury. The board shall make an annual report to the governor and to the Illinois pharmaceutical association of all moneys received and disbursed by them pursuant to this act. (As amended by act approved June 4, 1889; in force July 1, 1889.)

SEC. 12. Any person not being, or having in his employ, a registered pharmacist, within the meaning of this act, who shall, sixty days after this act takes effect, keep a pharmacy, or store for retailing or compounding medicines, or who shall take, use, or exhibit the title of a registered pharmacist, shall, for each and every such offense, be liable to a penalty of fifty dollars. Any registered pharmacist who shall permit the compounding and dispensing of prescriptions, or the vending of drugs, medicines, or poisons in his store or place of business, except under the supervision of a registered pharmacist, or except by a "registered assistant" pharmacist, or any pharmacist or "registered assistant," who, while continuing in business, shall fail or neglect to procure his annual registration, or any person who shall willfully make any false representation to procure registration for himself or any other person, shall, for every such offense, be liable to a penalty of fifty dollars: *Provided*, That nothing in this act shall apply to nor in any manner interfere with the business of any physician, or prevent him from supplying to his patients such articles as may seem to him proper, nor with the making or vending of patent or proprietary medicines, or medicines placed in sealed packages, with the name of the contents and of the pharmacist or physician by whom prepared or compounded, nor with the sale of the usual domestic remedies by retail dealers, nor with the exclusively wholesale business of any dealers, except as hereinafter provided: *And provided further*, That no part of this section shall be so construed as to give the right to any physician to furnish any intoxicating liquor as a beverage, on prescription or otherwise.

SEC. 13. No person shall add to or remove from any drug, medicine, chemical or pharmaceutical preparation any ingredient or material for the purpose of adulteration or substitution, or which shall deteriorate the quality, commercial value, or medicinal effect, or which shall alter the nature or composition of such drug, medicine, chemical or pharmaceutical preparation so that it will not correspond to the recognized tests of identity or purity. Any person who shall thus wilfully adulterate or alter, or cause to be adulterated or altered, or shall sell or offer for sale any such adulterated or altered drug, medicine, chemical or pharmaceutical preparation, or any person who shall substitute, or cause to be substituted, one material for another, with the intention to defraud or deceive the purchaser, shall be guilty of a misdemeanor, and be liable to prosecution under this act. If convicted, he shall be liable to all the costs of the action and all the expenses incurred by the board of pharmacy in connection therewith, and for the first offense be liable to a fine of not less than fifty dollars nor more than one hundred dollars, and for each subsequent offense a fine of not less than seventy-five nor more than one hundred and fifty dollars. On complaint being entered, the board of pharmacy is hereby empowered to employ an analyst or chemist expert, whose duty it shall be to examine into the so-claimed adulteration, substitution, or alteration, and report upon the result of his investigation; and if said report justify such action, the board shall duly cause the prosecution of the offender, as provided in this law.

SEC. 14. No person shall sell at retail any poisons commonly recognized as such, and especially aconite, arsenic, belladonna, biniodide of mercury, carbolic acid, chloral hydrate, chloroform, conium, corrosive sublimate, creosote, croton oil, cyanide of potassium, digitalis, hydrocyanic acid, laudanum, morphine, nux vomica, oil of bitter almonds, opium, oxalic acid, strychnine, sugar of lead, sulphate of zinc, white precipitate, red precipitato, without affixing to the box, bottle, vessel, or package containing the same, and to the wrapper or cover thereof, a label bearing the name of the article and the word "poison," distinctly shown, with the name and place of business of the seller; who shall not deliver any of said poisons to any person under the age of fifteen years, nor shall he deliver any of said poisons to any person without satisfying himself that such poison is to be used for a legitimate purpose: *Provided*, That nothing herein contained shall apply to the dispensing of physicians' prescriptions of any of the poisons aforesaid. Any person failing to comply with the requirements of this section shall be liable to a penalty of five dollars for each and every such offense.

SEC. 15. All suits for the recovery of the several penalties prescribed in this act shall be prosecuted in the name of the "People of the State of Illinois," in any court having jurisdiction; and it shall be the duty of the State's attorney of the county where such offense is committed to prosecute all persons violating the provisions of this act, upon proper complaint being made. All penalties collected under the provisions of this act shall inure, one-half to the board of pharmacy, and the remainder to the school fund of the county in which the suit was prosecuted and judgment obtained.

Original act approved May 30, 1881.
Amendments approved June 4, 1889.

## INDIANA.

Mr. Frank H. Carter, president of the Indiana State Pharmaceutical Association, writes, April 11, 1893:

We have no pharmacy law in Indiana.

## INDIAN TERRITORY.

Has no laws on the subject.

## IOWA.

### PHARMACY LAW.

#### CHAPTER 75.

ACTS OF THE EIGHTEENTH GENERAL ASSEMBLY AS AMENDED BY CHAPTER 137, ACTS OF THE NINETEENTH GENERAL ASSEMBLY; CHAPTER 83, ACTS OF THE TWENTY-FIRST GENERAL ASSEMBLY; CHAPTERS 71, 81, AND 106, ACTS OF TWENTY-SECOND GENERAL ASSEMBLY, AND CHAPTER 36, ACTS OF THE TWENTY-THIRD GENERAL ASSEMBLY, TO REGULATE THE SALE OF MEDICINES AND POISONS.

AN ACT to regulate the practice of pharmacy and the sale of medicines and poisons.

*Be it enacted by the General Assembly of the State of Iowa:*

SECTION 1. That from and after the passage of this act it shall be unlawful for any person, not a registered pharmacist within the meaning of this act, to conduct any pharmacy, drug store, apothecary shop or store for the purpose of retailing, compounding, or dispensing medicines or poisons, and any person violating the provisions of this section shall be liable to pay a penalty of five dollars for each day of such violation and cost of prosecution. Suits brought to recover any of the penalties provided for in this act (chapter 71, laws of 1888), or the acts to which it is amendatory, shall be instituted in the name of the State of Iowa by the county attorney, or under the direction and by the authority of the commissioners of pharmacy for the State of Iowa. In all cases brought under this act (chapter 71, Laws of 1888), or the acts to which it is amendatory, the prosecution need not prove that the defendant has not the required pharmacy certificate of registration; if the defendant has such certificate he must produce it.

SEC. 2. That it shall be unlawful for the proprietor of any store or pharmacy to allow any person except a registered pharmacist to compound or dispense the prescriptions of physicians, or to retail or dispense poisons for medical use, except as an aid to, and under the supervision of, a registered pharmacist. Any person violating the provisions of this section shall be deemed guilty of a misdemeanor, and, on conviction thereof, shall be liable to a fine of not less than twenty-five dollars, nor more than one hundred dollars, for each and every such offense.

SEC. 3. The governor, with the advice of the executive council, shall appoint three persons from among the most competent pharmacists of the State, all of whom shall have been residents of the State for five years, and of at least five years' practical experience in their profession, who shall be known and styled as commissioners of pharmacy for the State of Iowa; one of whom shall hold his office for one year, one for two years, and the other for three years, and each until his successor shall be appointed and qualified; and each year thereafter another commissioner shall be so appointed for three years, and until a successor be appointed and qualified. If a vacancy occur in said Commission, another shall be appointed, as aforesaid, to fill the unexpired term thereof. Said commissioners shall have power to make by-laws and all necessary regulations for the proper fulfillment of their duties under this act, without expense to the State, except that the secretary of state is authorized to furnish said commissioners with stationery and blanks necessary for their office. And said commissioners are authorized to administer oaths and take and certify the acknowledgments of instruments in writing.

SEC. 4. The commissioners of pharmacy shall register, in a suitable book, the names and places of residence of all persons to whom they issue certificates, and dates thereof. Druggists and pharmacists who were registered without examination shall not forfeit their registration when they have voluntarily sold, parted with, or severed their connections with the drug business for a period of two years at the place designated in certificate of registration. Should such party wish to reengage in the practice of pharmacy, he will not be required to be registered by examination as per section 5: *Provided*, That registered pharmacists who remove to another locality and reëngage in the practice of pharmacy within a period of two years, and have paid to the commission of pharmacy the sum of one dollar on or before the 22d day of March of each year, as provided in this chapter, such registered pharmacists shall not be required to register by examination, but his former registration shall be in full force and effect. Every registered pharmacist who desires to continue his profession shall, on or before the 22d day of March of each year, pay to the commission of pharmacy the sum of one dollar, for which he shall receive a renewal of his certificate, unless his name has been stricken from the register for violation of law. It shall be the duty of each registered pharmacist, before changing the locality as designated in his certificate of registration, to notify the secretary of the commission of pharmacy of his new place of business, and for recording the same and certification thereto the secretary shall be entitled to receive fifty cents for each certificate. It shall be the duty of every registered pharmacist to conspicuously post his certificate of registration in his place of business. Any person continuing in business, who shall fail or neglect to procure his annual renewal of registration, or who shall change his place of business without complying with this section, or who shall fail to conspicuously post his certificate of registration in his place of business, shall for each such offense be liable to a fine of ten dollars for each calendar month during which he is so delinquent.

SEC. 5. That the said commissioners of pharmacy shall, upon application, and at such time and place and in such manner as they may determine, examine, either by a schedule of questions to be answered and subscribed to under oath, or orally, each and every person who shall desire to conduct the business of selling at retail, compounding or dispensing drugs, medicines, or chemicals for medicinal use, or compounding or dispensing physicians' prescriptions as pharmacists, and if a majority of said commissioners shall be satisfied that said person is competent and fully qualified to conduct said business of compounding or dispensing drugs, medicines, or chemicals for medicinal use, or to compound or dispense physicians' prescriptions, they shall enter the name of such person as a registered pharmacist in the book provided for in section 4 of this act; and all graduates in pharmacy, having a diploma from an incorporated college or school of pharmacy that requires a practical experience in pharmacy of not less than four years before granting a diploma, shall be entitled to have their names registered as pharmacists by said commissioners of pharmacy without examination.

SEC. 6. That the commissioners of pharmacy shall be entitled to demand and receive from each person whom they register and furnish a certificate as a registered pharmacist, without examination, the sum of two dollars; and from each and every person whom they examine orally, or whose answers to a schedule of questions are returned subscribed to under oath, the sum of five dollars, which shall be in full for all services. And in case the examination of said person shall prove defective and unsatisfactory, and his name not be registered, he shall be permitted to present himself for reëxamination within any period not exceeding twelve months next thereafter, and no charge shall be made for such reëxamination.

SEC. 7. Every registered pharmacist shall be held responsible for the quality of all drugs, chemicals, and medicines he may sell or dispense, with the exception of those sold in the original packages of the manufacturer, and also those known as patent medicines, and should he knowingly, intentionally, and fraudulently adulterate, or cause to be adulterated, such drugs, chemicals, or medical preparations he shall be deemed guilty of a misdemeanor, and, upon conviction thereof, be liable to a penalty not exceeding one hundred dollars, and in addition thereto his name be stricken from the register.

SEC. 8. Pharmacists whose certificates of registration are in full force and effect shall have the sole right to keep and to sell, under such regulations as have been or may be established from time to time by the commissioners of pharmacy, all medicines and poisons excepting intoxicating liquors.

SEC. 9. It shall be unlawful for any person, from and after the passage of this act, to retail any poisons enumerated in schedules A and B, except as follows:

### SCHEDULE A.

Arsenic and its preparations, corosive sublimate, white precipitate, red precipitate, biniodide of mercury, cyanide of potassium, hydrocyanic acid, strychnia, and all other poisonous vegetable alkaloids and their salts, essential oil of bitter almonds, opium and its preparations, except paregoric and other preparations of opium containing less than two grains to the ounce.

### SCHEDULE B.

Aconite, belladonna, colchicum, conium, nux vomica, henbane, savin, ergot, cotton root, cantharides, creosote, digitalis, and their pharmaceutical preparations; croton oil, chloroform, chloral hydrate, sulphate of zinc, mineral acids, carbolic acid and oxalic acid, without distinctly labeling the box, vessel, or paper in which the said poison is contained, and also the outside wrapper or cover, with the name of the article, the word "poison," and the name and place of business of the seller. Nor shall it be lawful for any person to sell or deliver any poison enumerated in schedules A and B unless, upon due inquiry, it be found that the purchaser is aware of its poisonous character, and represents that it is to be used for a legitimate purpose. Nor shall it be lawful for any registered pharmacist to sell any poisons included in schedule A without, before delivering the same to the purchaser, causing an entry to be made, in a book kept for that purpose, stating the date of sale, the name and the address of the purchaser, the name of the poison sold, the purpose for which it is represented by the purchaser to be required, and the name of the dispenser, such book to be always open for inspection by the proper authorities, and to be preserved for at least five years. The provisions of this section shall not apply to the dispensing of poisons, in not unusual quantities or doses, upon the prescriptions of practitioners of medicine. Nor shall it be lawful for any licensed or registered druggist or pharmacist to retail, or sell, or give away, any alcoholic liquors or compounds as a beverage, and any violations of the provisions of this section shall make the owner or principal of said store or pharmacy liable to a fine of not less than twenty-five dollars, and not more than one hundred dollars, to be collected in the usual manner; and, in addition thereto, for repeated violations of this section, his name shall be stricken from the register.

SEC. 10. Any itinerant vender of any drug, nostrum, ointment, or appliance of any kind, intended for the treatment of diseases or injury, who shall, by writing or printing, or any other method, publicly profess to cure or treat diseases, or injury, or deformity, by any drug, nostrum, or manipulation, or other expedient, shall pay a license of one hundred dollars per annum, to be paid to the treasurer of the commission of pharmacy. Whereupon the secretary of said commission shall issue such license for one year. Any person violating this section shall be deemed guilty of a misdemeanor, and shall, upon conviction, pay a fine of not less than one hundred nor more than two hundred dollars. All moneys received for license to be reported to the auditor of State. The sum of two thousand dollars per year, or as much thereof as may be necessary, is hereby appropriated out of the moneys so received for licenses for the expenses of said commission; all exceeding said amount to be paid into the State treasury.

SEC. 11. That any person who shall procure, or attempt to procure, registration for himself or for another under this act, by making, or causing to be made, any false representations, shall be deemed guilty of a misdemeanor, and shall, upon conviction thereof, be liable to a penalty of not less than twenty-five nor more than one hundred dollars, and the name of the person so fraudulently registered shall be stricken from the register. Any person not a registered pharmacist, as provided for in this act, who shall conduct a store, pharmacy, or place for retailing, compounding or dispensing drugs, medicines, or chemicals, for medicinal use, or for compounding or dispensing physicians' prescriptions, or who shall take, use, or exhibit the title of registered pharmacist, shall be deemed guilty of a misdemeanor, and, upon conviction thereof, shall be liable to a penalty of not less than fifty dollars nor more than two hundred dollars.

SEC. 12. Physicians dispensing their own prescriptions only are not required to be registered pharmacists: *Provided*, That nothing in this act (chapter 83, Laws 1886) shall prevent any person not a registered pharmacist or not holding a permit from keeping and selling proprietary medicines, and such other domestic remedies as do not include any intoxicating liquors or poisons, nor from selling concentrated lye and potash: *Provided, however*, That if any person sell or deliver said concentrated lye or potash without having the word "poison" and the true name thereof written or printed upon a label attached to the vial, box, or parcel containing the same, shall be punished by imprisonment in the county jail not more than thirty days, or by fine not exceeding one hundred dollars, but they shall not be compelled to register the sales of said lye and potash as required by section 4038, Code of 1873.

SEC. 13. This act, being deemed of immediate importance, shall take effect from and after its publication in the Iowa State Register and Iowa State Leader, newspapers published at Des Moines, Iowa.

SEC. 14. All acts and parts of acts in conflict with this act are hereby repealed.

Original act, chapter 75, approved March 22, 1880, published in the Iowa State Leader, March 27, 1880, and in the Iowa State Register, March 31, 1880.

NOTES.

Chapter 137, approved March 17, 1882, published in the Iowa State Leader and the Iowa State Register, March, 1882.

Chapter 83, approved April 17, 1886, published in the Iowa State Leader and the Iowa State Register, April 8, 1886.

Chapter 71, approved April 12, 1888, published in the Iowa State Register and Des Moines Leader, April 13, 1888.

Chaper 81, approved March 28, 1888, published in the Iowa State Register and Des Moines Leader, March 31, 1888.

Chapter 106, approved April 12, 1888, published in the Iowa State Register and Des Moines Leader, April 19, 1888.

Chapter 35, approved April 18, 1890, published in the Des Moines Leader, April 22, 1890, and in the Iowa State Register, April 23, 1890.

Chapter 36, approved May 15, 1890, having no publication clause, took effect July 4, 1890.

### ABSTRACT OF THE PHARMACY LAW.

Chapter 75 of the eighteenth general assembly, first enactment, March 22, 1890, section 1, in force as amended by section 21, chapter 71, twenty-second general assembly.

Section 2, in force.

Section 3 is in force as amended by section 1, chapter 83, twenty-first general assembly.

Section 4 is in force as amended by section 1, chapter 137, nineteenth general assembly; section 1, chapter 106, twenty-second general assembly, section 22, chapter 71, twenty-second general assembly; and section 1, chapter 36, twenty-third general assembly.

Section 5 is in force.

Section 6 is in force.

Section 7 is in force.

Section 8, substitute enacted by section 2, chapter 83, twenty-first general assembly, and as amended by section 20, chapter 71, twenty-second general assembly.

Section 9 is in force.

Section 10 is in force as amended by section 2, chapter 137, nineteenth general assembly, and section 3, chapter 83, twenty-first general assembly.

Section 11 is in force as amended by section 3, chapter 137, nineteenth general assembly.

Section 12, substitute enacted by section 4, chapter 83, twenty-first general assembly.

Section 13, publication clause.

Section 14, repealing clause.

### CHAPTER 71.—TO REGULATE THE SALE OF INTOXICATING LIQUORS.

AN ACT to provide for and regulate the sale of intoxicating liquors for necessary purposes, and to make more efficient the laws for the suppression of intemperance, and to repeal sections 1524, 1526, 1527, 1528, 1529, 1530, 1531, 1532, 1533, 1534, 1535, 1536, 1537, and 1538 of the code of 1873, as amended by chapter 143, of the acts of the Twentieth General Assembly, and all that part of section two (2) chapter eighty-three (83), acts of the Twenty-first general assembly, after the words "medicines and poisons" in the fifth line thereof; and to amend sections 1 and 4, chapter 75, acts of the Eighteenth General Assembly, and to provide penalties and proceedings for violations of the provisions thereof.

*Be it enacted by the General Assembly of the State of Iowa:*

[NOTE.—Sections 1, 2, 3, 4, 5, 6, 7, 8, 9, 10, 11, 12, 13, 14, 15, 16, 17, 18, and 19 of this chapter have been repealed by chapter 35, laws of 1890.]

SEC. 20. That sections 1524, 1526, 1527, 1528, 1529, 1530, 1531, 1532, 1533, 1534, 1535, 1536, 1537, and 1538 of the code of 1873, as amended by chapter 143 of the acts of the

Twentieth General Assembly, and all that part of section two (2), chapter eighty-three (83), acts of the Twenty-first General Assembly, after the words "medicines and poisons" in the fifth line thereof, be, and the same is hereby, repealed, and by inserting after the word "poison" in the fifth line of section two, chapter eighty-three, acts of the Twenty-first General Assembly, the following words: "excepting intoxicating liquors:" *Provided*, That nothing in this act shall be construed to abate any action or proceeding now pending in any court in this State for a violation of the provisions of the sections hereby repealed, or to operate to bar any prosecutions hereafter brought for any such violations committed prior to the passage and taking effect of this act.

SEC. 21. That section one, chapter 75, of the acts of the Eighteenth General Assembly be, and the same is hereby, amended by striking out the words "for medical use, except as hereinafter provided," at the end of said section and inserting in lieu thereof the words, "and any person violating the provisions of this section shall be liable to pay a penalty of five dollars for each day of such violation, and cost of prosecution. Suits brought to recover any of the penalties provided for in this act or the acts to which it is amendatory shall be instituted in the name of the State of Iowa by the county attorney or under the direction and by the authority of the commissioners of pharmacy for the State of Iowa. In all cases brought under this act or the acts to which it is amendatory, the prosecution need not prove that the defendant has not the required pharmacy certificate of registration; if the defendant has such certificate he must produce it."

SEC. 22. That section 4, chapter 75, of the acts of the Eighteenth General Assembly be, and the same is hereby, amended, by striking out the words "a duplicate of which is to be kept in the secretary of State's office," in the second and third lines of said section.

SEC. 23. This act being deemed of immediate importance shall take effect and be in force from and after its publication in the Iowa State Register and Des Moines Leader, newspapers published in Des Moines, Iowa.

Approved April 12, 1888.

CHAPTER 81.—TO AMEND CHAPTER 83, ACTS OF TWENTY-FIRST GENERAL ASSEMBLY. SALE OF POISONS.

AN ACT to amend chapter 83, acts of the Twenty-first General Assembly, relating to the sale of poisons.

*Be it enacted by the General Assembly of the State of Iowa:*

SECTION 1. That section 4, chapter 83, acts of the Twenty-first General Assembly, be, and the same is hereby, amended by adding to the end thereof the following:

"Nor from selling concentrated lye and potash: *Provided, however*, That if any person sell or deliver said concentrated lye or potash without having the word 'poison' and the true name thereof written or printed upon a label attached to the vial, box, or parcel containing the same, shall be punished by imprisonment in the county jail not more than thirty days, or by fine not exceeding one hundred dollars, but they shall not be compelled to register the sales of said lye and potash as required by section 4038, code of 1873.

SEC. 2. This act being deemed of immediate importance, shall be in full force and effect on and after its publication in the Iowa State Register and Daily Des Moines Leader, newspapers published in Des Moines, Iowa.

Approved March 28, 1888.

CHAPTER 106.—REMOVAL FROM ONE PLACE TO ANOTHER OF REGISTERED PHARMACISTS.

AN ACT to amend section 1, chapter 137, laws of the Nineteenth (19th) General Assembly, relating to registered pharmacists.

*Be it enacted by the General Assembly of the State of Iowa:*

SECTION 1. That section one (1) chapter one hundred and thirty-seven (137), laws of the Nineteenth General Assembly, be amended by adding to said section after the number "five" (5), in the eleventh line, the following : "*Provided*, That registered pharmacists who remove to another locality, and reëngage in the practice of pharmacy within a period of two years, and have paid to the commission of pharmacy the sum of one dollar on or before the 22d day of March of each year, as provided in this chapter. Such registered pharmacist shall not be required to register by examination, but his former registration shall be in full force and effect."

Sec. 2. This act being deemed of immediate importance shall take effect and be in force from and after its publication in the Iowa State Register and Iowa State Leader, newspapers published at Des Moines, Iowa.

Approved April 12, 1888.

CHAPTER 36, LAWS OF 1890.—RELATING TO PHARMACISTS REGISTERED WITHOUT EXAMINATION.

AN ACT to amend section one (1) of chapter one hundred and thirty-seven (137), acts of the Nineteenth (19th) General Assembly, relating to pharmacists registered without examination.

*Be it enacted by the General Assembly of the State of Iowa:*

SECTION 1. That section one (1) of chapter one hundred and thirty-seven (137), acts of the Nineteenth (19th) General Assembly, be amended by inserting after the word "examination" in the fifth (5th) line the words "shall not," and by striking out the words "who has thus forfeited his registration" in the ninth (9th) line, and by striking out the word "is" in the tenth (10th) line and inserting in lieu thereof the words "will not be."

Approved May 15, 1890.

NOTE.—The above act having no publication clause took effect July 4, 1890.

CHAPTER 35, LAWS OF 1890.—TO REGULATE THE KEEPING AND SALE OF INTOXICATING LIQUORS.

AN ACT to provide for and regulate the keeping and sale of intoxicating liquors for lawful purposes, and to repeal sections 1, 2, 3, 4, 5, 6, 7, 8, 9, 10, 11, 12, 13, 14, 15, 16, 17, 18, and 19, of chapter 71, laws of the Twenty-second General Assembly.

*Be it enacted by the General Assembly of the State of Iowa:*

SECTION 1. That sections 1, 2, 3, 4, 5, 6, 7, 8, 9, 10, 11, 12, 13, 14, 15, 16, 17, 18, and 19, of chapter 71, laws of the Twenty-second General Assembly, be, and the same are hereby, repealed, and the following enacted in lieu thereof:

SEC. 2. That after this act takes effect no person shall manufacture for sale, sell, keep for sale, give away, exchange, barter, or dispense any intoxicating liquor, for any purpose whatever, otherwise than as provided in this act. Persons holding permits, as herein provided, shall be authorized to sell and dispense intoxicating liquors for pharmaceutical and medical purposes, and alcohol for specified chemical and mechanical purposes, and wine for sacramental purposes and to sell to registered pharmacists and manufacturers of proprietary medicines, for use in compounding medicines, and to permit-holders for use and resale by them, for the purposes authorized by this act, but for no other purposes whatever; and all permits must be procured, as hereinafter provided, from the district court of the proper county at any term thereof after this act takes effect, and a permit to buy and sell intoxicating liquors, when so procured shall continue in force until revoked according to law: *Provided, further*, That this section shall not be construed to prevent licensed physicians from dispensing in good faith such liquors as medicine to patients actually sick and under their treatment at the time of such dispensing: *Provided, further*, That in case of death or other disability of any registered pharmacist the administrator, guardian, or legal representative of such pharmacist may continue such business subject to the provisions of this act through the agency of any reputable registered pharmacist conditioned upon there being first obtained the approval of the district court or clerk thereof: *Provided, further,* That before entering upon such duties such party or person shall file with the clerk of said court a bond as herein provided, to be approved by the clerk of said court.

SEC. 3. Notice of an application for a permit must be published for three consecutive weeks in a newspaper regularly published and printed in the English language, and of general circulation in the city or town where the applicant proposes to keep and sell intoxicating liquors, or if there be no newspaper regularly published in such city or town such publication shall be made in one of the official papers of the county, the last of which publication shall be not less than ten days nor more than twenty days before the first day of the term; and state the name of the applicant, with the firm name under which he is doing business, the purpose of the application, the particular location, or the place where the applicant proposes to keep and sell liquors, and that the petition provided for in the next section will be on file in the clerk's office at least ten days before the first day of the term, naming it, when the application will be made, and a copy thereof shall be served personally upon the county attorney in the same manner and time as required for service of original notices in the district court.

SEC. 4. Applications for permits shall be made by petitions signed and sworn to by the applicant and filed in the office of the clerk of the district court of the proper county at least ten days before the first day of the term, which petition shall state the applicant's name, place of residence, in what business he is then engaged, and in what business he has been engaged for two years previous to filing the petition; the place, particularly describing it, where the business of buying and selling liquor is to be conducted; that he is a citizen of the United States and of the State of Iowa; and that he is a registered pharmacist and now is, and for the last six months has been, lawfully conducting a pharmacy in the township or town wherein he proposes to sell intoxicating liquors under the permit applied for, and as the proprietor of such pharmacy that he has been adjudged guilty of violating the law relating to intoxicating liquors within the last year next preceding his application; and is not the keeper of a hotel, eating house, saloon, restaurant, or place of public amusement; that he is not addicted to the use of intoxicating liquors as a beverage, and that he desires a permit to purchase, keep, and sell such liquors for lawful purposes only. And every applicant who has at any time taken out a permit under this act which said permit has been revoked, shall, if he again apply for a permit, file with such application the further statement under oath, that he has not within the last two years next preceding his application, been knowingly engaged, employed, or interested in the unlawful manufacture, sale, or keeping for sale of intoxicating liquors: " *Provided, further,* When a pharmacist has procured a permit, and by reason of the expiration of his lease, or for any other good reason, he desires to change his locality to another place in the same township, town, or ward, the court may grant to him on his petition, the right to continue business under his permit in the same township, town, or ward in which the permit is granted."

SEC. 5. This permit shall issue only on condition that the applicant shall execute to the State of Iowa a bond in the penal sum of one thousand dollars with good and sufficient sureties to be approved by the clerk of the court, conditioned that he will well and truly observe and obey the laws of Iowa, now or hereafter in force, in relation to the sale of intoxicating liquors, that he will pay all fines, penalties, damages, and costs that may be assessed or recovered against him for a violation of such laws during the term for which said permit is granted. The said bond shall be deposited with the county auditor, and suit shall be brought thereon at any time by the county attorney, or any person for whose benefit the same is given, and in case the conditions thereof or any of them shall be violated, the principals and sureties therein shall be jointly and severally liable for all civil damages, costs, and judgments that may be obtained against the principal in any civil action brought by a wife, child, parent, guardian, employer, or other person, under the provisions of section fifteen hundred and fifty-six, fifteen hundred and fifty-seven, and fifteen hundred and fifty-eight of the code of Iowa, as the same is amended and now in force, and section twelve, chapter sixty-six, acts of the Twenty-first general assembly of the State of Iowa. The clear proceeds of all other money collected for breaches of such bond shall go to the school fund of the county. Said bond shall be approved by the clerk of the district court under the rules and laws applicable to the approval of official bonds. If at any time the sureties or any of them on said bond shall become insolvent or be deemed insufficient by the clerk of the district court said clerk shall require a new bond to be executed within a time to be fixed by him, and a failure of the person holding such permit to execute such new and sufficient bond within the time fixed by said clerk therefor shall cause said permit to become null and void. If the application for the permit is granted it shall not issue until the applicant shall make and subscribe an oath before the clerk, which shall be indorsed upon the bond to the effect and tenor following:

"I, ———— ————, do solemnly swear (or affirm) that I will well and truly perform all and singular the conditions of the within bond, and keep and perform the trust confided in me to purchase, keep, and sell intoxicating liquors. I will not sell, give, or furnish to any person any intoxicating liquors otherwise than as provided by law, and, especially, I will not sell or furnish any intoxicating liquors to any person who is not known to me personally, or duly identified; nor to any minor, intoxicated person or persons who are in the habit of becoming intoxicated; and I will make true, full, and accurate returns of all certificates and requests made to or received by me as required by law; and said returns shall show every sale and delivery of such liquors made by or for me during the months embraced therein, and the true signatures to every request received and granted; and such returns shall show all the intoxicating liquors sold or delivered to any and every person as returned."

Upon taking said oath and filing bond as hereinbefore provided, the clerk shall issue to him a permit authorizing him to keep and sell intoxicating liquors as in this act provided; and every permit so granted, shall specify the building, giving the street and number, or location in which intoxicating liquors may be sold by virtue of the same, and the length of time the same shall be in force.

SEC. 6. No application for a permit shall be considered or acted upon by the court until the requisite notice has been given and petition filed as provided by this act and each is in form and substance such as require. On the first day of the term, having ascertained that the application is properly presented the court shall proceed to hear the application, unless objection thereto be made, in which case the court shall appoint a day during the term, but not later, when the same will be heard; and in doing so shall consider the convenience of the court, and the interested parties and their counsel so far as the state of the business and the necessities of the case will permit.

If unavoidable causes prevent a hearing during the regular time allotted to the term, the same shall be heard and disposed of in vacation by the judge as soon as practicable thereafter. The county attorney or other counsel, or any five citizens, may in person or by counsel appear and resist the application. Any remonstrance or objection thereto must be in writing and filed on or before noon of the first day of the said term or by such later time as may be fixed by the court, and before the date fixed for hearing, and such remonstrance shall state specifically the objection thereto. And whether resisted or objection be made or not the court shall not grant the permit until it shall first be made to appear by competent evidence that the applicant is possessed of the character and qualifications requisite, is worthy of confidence and to receive the trust and will be likely to execute the same with fidelity; and that the statements made in his application are all and singular true, and, considering the population of the locality and the reasonable necessities and convenience of the people such permit is proper. If the application is resisted the court or judge shall hear controversy upon the petitions, remonstrances, and objections, and the evidence offered, and grant or refuse such permit as the public good may require. If there be more than one permit applied for in the same locality they shall all be heard at the same time, unless for good cause otherwise directed, and the court may grant or refuse any or all of the applications as will best subserve the public interest.

SEC. 7. Permits granted under this act shall be deemed trusts reposed in the recipients thereof, and may be revoked upon sufficient showing by order of the court or judge thereof. Complaint may be presented at any time to the district court, or one of the judges thereof, which shall be in writing and signed and sworn to by three citizens of the county in which the permit was granted, and a copy of such complaint shall, with a notice in writing of the time and place of hearing be served on the accused five days before the hearing, and if the complaint is sufficient, and the accused appear and deny the same, the court or judge shall proceed without delay, unless continued for cause, to hear and determine the controversy, but if continued or appealed at the instance of the permit holder, his permit to buy and sell liquors, may, in the discretion of the court, be suspended pending the controversy. The complainant and accused may be heard in person, or by counsel, or both, and submit such proofs as may be offered by the parties; and if it shall appear upon such hearing that the accused has in any way abused the trust, or that liquors are sold by the accused or his employés in violation of law, or if it shall appear that any liquor has been sold or dispensed unlawfully or has been unlawfully obtained at said place from the holder of the permit or any employé assisting therein, or that he has in any proceeding, civil or criminal, since receiving his permit, been adjudged guilty of violating any of the provisions of this act or the acts for the suppression of intemperance, the court or judge shall by order revoke and set aside the permit; the papers and order in such case shall be immediately returned to and filed by the clerk of the court, if heard by the judge and the order entered of record as if made in court, and if in this or any other proceeding, civil or criminal, it shall be adjudged by the court or judge that any registered pharmacist, proprietor, or clerk who has been guilty of violating this act or the act for the suppression of intemperance and amendments thereto, by unlawfully manufacturing, selling, giving away, or unlawfully keeping with intend to sell intoxicating liquors, such adjudication may, in the discretion of the commissioners of pharmacy, if such violations are thereafter repeated, work a forfeiture of his certificate of registration. It shall be the duty of the clerk to forward to the commissioners of pharmacy such transcripts without charge therefor, as soon as practicable after final judgment or order.

SEC. 8. Registered pharmacists, who show themselves to be fit persons and who comply with all the requirements of this act, may be granted permits, and in any township where there is a registered pharmacist conducting a pharmacy and no pharmacist obtains a permit, if found necessary the court may grant a permit to one discreet person in such township not a pharmacist, but having all other qualifications requisite under this act, upon like notice and proceedings as pertain to permitted pharmacists and subject to the same liabilities, duties, obligations, and penalties.

SEC. 9. The clerk of the court granting the permit shall preserve as a part of the record and files of his office all petitions, bonds, and other papers pertaining to the granting or revocation of permits, and keep suitable books in which bonds and permits shall be recorded. The books shall be furnished by the county like other public records. Whether said permit be granted or refused, the applicant shall pay the costs incurred in the case, and when granted he shall make payment before any permit issue, except the court may tax the cost of any witnesses summoned by private persons resisting said application, and the fees for serving such subpœnas to such persons, when it is shown that such witnesses were summoned maliciously, or without probable cause to believe their evidence material. A fee of one dollar and fifty cents shall be taxed for the filing of the petition, and one dollar for entering the order of the court approving bond and granting said application, and witnesses shall be entitled to mileage and per diem as in other cases. And fees for serving notices and subpœnas shall be the same as in other cases in the district court.

SEC. 10. Before selling or delivering any intoxicating liquors to any person, a request must be printed or written, dated of the true date, stating the applicant is not a minor, and the residence of the signer, for whom and whose use the liquor is required, the amount and kind required, the actual purpose for which the request is made and for what use desired, and his or her true name and residence, and, where numbered, by street and number, if in a city, and that neither the applicant nor the person for whose use requested habitually uses intoxicating liquors as a beverage, and the request shall be signed by the applicant by his own true name and signature, and attested by the permit-holder who receives and fills the request by his own true name and signature in his own handwriting. But the request shall be refused, notwithstanding the statement made, unless the permit-holder has reason to believe said statement to be true, and in no case unless the permit-holder filling it personally knows the person applying, that he is not a minor, that he is not intoxicated, and that he is not in the habit of using intoxicating liquors as a beverage; or, if the applicant is not so personally known to the permit-holder, before filling the said order or delivering the liquor he shall require identification, and the statement of a reliable and trustworthy person, of good character and habits, known personally to him, that the applicant is not a minor, and is not in the habit of using intoxicating liquors as a beverage, and is worthy of credit as to the truthfulness of the statements in the application, and this statement shall be signed by the witness in his own true name and handwriting, stating his residence correctly.

SEC. 11. On or before the 15th of January, March, May, July, September, and November of each year each permit-holder shall make full returns to the county auditor of all requests filled by him and his clerks during the two preceding months, and accompanying the same with a written or printed oath duly taken and subscribed before the county auditor or notary public, which shall be in the following form, to wit: "I, ........................, being duly sworn, on oath state that the requests for liquors herewith returned are all that were received and filled at my pharmacy (or place of business) under my permit during the months of ———, 18——; that I have carefully preserved the same and that they were filled up, signed and attested at the date shown thereon, as provided by law; that said requests were filled by delivering the quantity and kind of liquors required, and that no liquors have been sold or dispensed under color of my permit during said months except as shown by the requests herewith returned, and that I have faithfully observed and complied with the conditions of my bond and oath taken by me thereon endorsed and with all the laws relating to any duties in the premises."

Every permit-holder shall keep strict account of all liquors purchased or procured by him in a book kept for that purpose, which shall be subject at all times to the inspection of the commissioners of pharmacy and the county attorney, and any grand juror, sheriff, or justice of the peace of the county, and such books shall show of whom such liquors were purchased or procured, the amount and kind of liquors purchased or procured, the date of receipt and amount sold, also the amount on hand of each kind for each two months; such book shall be produced by the party keeping the same, to be used as evidence on the trial of any prosecution against him or against liquors alleged to have been seized from him or his house, on notice duly served that the same will be required as evidence; and at the same time he returns requests to the county auditor he shall file a statement of such account with such auditor, except that the items of sales need not be embraced therein, but the aggregate amount of each kind shall be, and such statement shall be verified before the county auditor or a notary public. All forms necessary to carry out the provisions of this act not otherwise provided for shall be as may be provided by the commissioners of pharmacy.

SEC. 12. Every permit-holder or his clerk under this act shall be subject to all the penalties, forfeitures, and judgments and may be prosecuted by all the proceedings and actions, criminal and civil, and whether at law or in equity, provided for or authorized by the laws now or hereafter in force, for any violation of this act and the act for the suppression of intemperance and any law regulating the sale of intoxicating liquors and by any or all of such proceedings applicable to complaints against such permit-holder; and the permit shall not shield any person who abuses the trust imposed by it or violates the laws aforesaid, and in case of conviction in any proceeding civil or criminal all the liquors in possession of the permit-holder may by order of the court be destroyed. On the trial of any action or proceeding against any person for manufacturing, selling, giving away, or keeping with intent to sell intoxicating liquors in violation of law, or for any failure to comply with the conditions or duties imposed by this act, the requests for liquors and returns made to the auditor as herein required, the quantity and kinds of liquors sold or kept, purchased or disposed of, the purpose for which liquors were obtained by or from him and for which they were used, the character and habits of sobriety or otherwise, shall be competent evidence and may be considered so far as applicable to the particular case with any other recognized, competent, and material facts and circumstances bearing on the issues involved in determining the ultimate facts. In any suit, prosecution, or proceedings for violations of this act or the acts for the suppression of intemperance, and acts amendatory thereof, the court may compel the production in evidence of any books or papers required by this act to be kept, and may compel any permit-holder, his clerk, or any person who has purchased liquors of either of them, to appear and give evidence, and the claim that any such testimony or evidence will tend to criminate the person giving such evidence shall not excuse such person or witness from testifying or producing such books or papers in evidence; but such oral evidence shall not be used against such person or witness, on the trial of any criminal proceeding against him. Any number of distinct violations of this act may be charged in one indictment or information in different counts and all tried in the same action, the jury specifying the counts, if any, on which the defendant is found guilty.

SEC. 13. Registered pharmacists, conducting pharmacies and not holding permits, and manufacturers of proprietary medicines are hereby authorized to purchase of permit-holders intoxicating liquors (not including malt) for the purpose of compounding medicines, tinctures, and extracts that can not be used as a beverage. Such purchasers shall keep a record of uses to which the same are devoted, giving the kind and quantity so used.

And on or before the 15th day of January, March, May, July, September, and November of each year they shall make and file with the county auditor sworn reports for the two preceding calendar months, giving full and true statements of the quantity and kinds of such liquors purchased and used, the uses to which the same have been devoted. The commissioners of pharmacy are hereby empowered to make such further rules and regulations with respect to the purchase, use, and keeping of such liquors as they may deem proper for the prevention of the abuses of the trusts reposed in such purchasers, and if the said registered pharmacist sell, barter, give away, exchange or in any manner dispose of said liquors, or use the same for any purpose other than authorized in this section he shall, upon conviction before any district court thereof, be liable to all the penalties, prosecutions, and proceedings at law or in equity provided against persons selling without a permit, and upon any such conviction the clerk of the district court shall within ten days after said judgment or order transmit to the commissioners of pharmacy the certified record thereof, upon receipt of which the commission may strike his name from the list of pharmacists and cancel his certificate: *Provided*, That nothing herein contained shall be construed to authorize the manufacture or sale of any preparation or compound under any name, form, or device, which may be used as a beverage and which is intoxicating in its character.

SEC. 14. Every permit-holder is hereby authorized to ship to registered pharmacists and manufacturers of proprietary medicines intoxicating liquors to be used by them for the purposes authorized by this act.

And all railway transportation and express companies, and other common carriers, are authorized to receive and transport the same upon presentation of a certificate from the clerk of the district court of the county where the permit-holder resides that such person is permitted to ship intoxicating liquors, under the provisions of this act.

SEC. 15. A permit-holder may employ one or more registered pharmacists as clerks, to sell intoxicating liquors in conformity to the permit and provisions of this act, but in such case the acts of his clerks in conducting the business shall be deemed the acts of the permit-holder, who shall be liable therefor as if he had personally done the acts, and in making returns the verification of such requests as may have been received, attested, and filled by a clerk must be made by such clerk, and the clerk who transacted any of the business under the permit must join in the general oath required of the employer so far as relates to his own connection therewith. If for any cause a registered pharmacist who holds a permit shall cease to hold a valid and subsisting certificate of registration or renewal thereof his permit shall thereby be forfeited and be null and void.

SEC. 16. Any person holding a permit in force when this act takes effect may continue to purchase, keep, and sell intoxicating liquors (according to law) for the time provided in such permit, unless sooner revoked. But all such permits shall expire not later than January 1st, 1891.

SEC. 17. If any person shall be convicted of violating any of the provisions of this act or acts regulating the practice of pharmacy or any acts for the suppression of intemperance, or amendments thereto by reason of a prosecution by the commissioners of pharmacy, the clear proceeds of all fines so imposed and collected shall be paid into the county treasury of the proper county for the use of the school fund, and the commissioners of pharmacy shall be entitled to draw from the State treasury an amount not exceeding 50 per cent of the amount of the fines so collected, to be used solely in prosecutions instituted by them for failure to comply with the provisions of this act or of the acts regulating the practice of pharmacy. And the court or clerk thereof before whom any prosecution is instituted and prosecuted by the commissioners of pharmacy shall certify to the auditor of State all cases in which they have appeared as prosecutors, either in person or by their attorney, and the amount of fines imposed and collected in such cases. And the commissioners of pharmacy shall have the power to revoke the certificate of registration of pharmacists for repeated violations of this act. Said amount to be drawn from time to time upon the warrants of the State auditor, which shall issue for the payment of expenses actually incurred in said prosecution after said expenses shall have been audited by the executive council.

SEC. 18. If any person shall make any false or fictitious signature or sign any name other than his or her own to any paper required to be signed by this act or make any false statement in any paper or application signed to procure liquors under this act, the person so offending shall be deemed guilty of a misdemeanor, and, upon conviction thereof, shall be punished by a fine of not less than twenty (20) dollars nor more than one hundred (100) dollars and cost of prosecution, and shall be committed until said fine and costs are paid, or be imprisoned not less than ten or more than thirty days. If any permit holder or his clerk shall make false oath touching any matter required to be sworn to under the provisions of this act, the person so offending shall, upon conviction thereof, be punished as provided by law for perjury. If any person holding a permit under this law shall purchase or procure any intoxicating liquor otherwise than authorized by this act, or make any false return to the county auditor, or use any request for liquors for more than one sale, in any of such cases he shall be deemed guilty of a misdemeanor, and, upon conviction, punished accordingly.

SEC. 19. Nothing in this act shall be construed to abate any action or proceeding now pending in any court in this State for a violation of the provisions of the sections hereby repealed, or to operate to bar any prosecutions hereafter brought for any such violations committed prior to the passage and taking effect of this act.

SEC. 20. The superior courts of this State and the judges and clerks thereof shall have and exercise the same powers and duties as are in this act specified for district courts, their judges and clerks as to granting and revoking permits.

SEC. 21. This act being deemed of immediate importance shall take effect and be in force from and after its publication in the Iowa State Register and the Des Moines Leader, newspapers published in Des Moines, Iowa.

Approved April 18, 1890.

Published in the Des Moines Leader April 22, 1890, and in the Iowa State Register April 23, 1890.

## KANSAS.

### CHAPTER 150.—THE PHARMACY LAW.

AN ACT entitled "An act to prevent incompetent or unauthorized persons from engaging in the practice of pharmacy; also to regulate the sale of poisons and proprietary medicines; to prevent and punish the adulteration of drugs, medicines, medicinal preparations, and chemicals; and to create a board of pharmacy for the regulation of the practice of pharmacy in the State of Kansas."

*Be it enacted by the Legislature of the State of Kansas:*

SECTION 1. It shall hereafter be unlawful for any person within the State of Kansas to open or conduct any pharmacy or store for retailing, dispensing, or compounding medicines or poisons, unless such person be a registered pharmacist within the meaning of this act, or shall employ a registered pharmacist to conduct the same. And it shall be unlawful for any person to compound and sell at retail any medicines or poisons, or to compound and dispense any physicians' prescriptions, unless such person be a registered pharmacist, or a registered assistant pharmacist, within the meaning of this act, except as hereinafter provided. Any person violating the provisions of this section shall be deemed guilty of a misdemeanor, and upon conviction thereof shall be liable to a fine of not less than twenty-five dollars nor more than one hundred dollars for each and every such offense.

SEC. 2. Repealed.

SEC. 3. The board of pharmacy shall register in a suitable book, a duplicate of which shall be kept in the office of the secretary of State, the names and places of residence of all persons to whom they issue certificates, and the date thereof. A copy of the record of the board, or of any portion thereof certified by its secretary, shall be deemed lawful evidence in any court of this State.

SEC. 7. It shall be the duty or every registered pharmacist or assistant pharmacist, upon changing his place of business, forthwith to notify by letter the secretary of the board of pharmacy of such change, and to inclose a fee of fifty cents, upon receipt of which the secretary shall make the necessary alteration in his register. It shall also be the duty of every registered pharmacist or assistant pharmacist to notify by letter said secretary, on the first day of July in each year, whether he still continues practicing pharmacy at registered place of business. The secretary shall notify every person who shall not have notified the board as herein provided, and in case an answer, enclosing a fee of fifty cents, shall not be received by the secretary within thirty days, such name shall be stricken from the register: *Provided always,* That his name may be restored to the register on the payment to the secretary, within one year, of a fee of five dollars. It shall be the duty of the secretary of the board to erase from the registry the name of any registered pharmacist who may have died, removed from, or ceased to do business in this State, and to make all necessary alterations in the location of the person registered under this act. He shall publish annually a list of all persons that are duly registered as pharmacists and assistant pharmacists, a copy of which shall be mailed free to each and every registered pharmacist and assistant pharmacist in the State.

SEC. 8. Any person not entitled to registration under the preceding provisions and who may desire a certificate as registered pharmacist, shall apply for examination to the board of pharmacy, and shall pay the secretary of the board the sum of five dollars. If the board shall find that he has had a practical experience of four years in compounding physicians' prescriptions in the general duties of pharmacy and is otherwise duly qualified, they shall duly register him and issue him a certificate as registered pharmacist. In case of failure to pass a satisfactory examination, a second examination may be granted within six months without further payment.

SEC. 9. Repealed.

SEC. 10. Every proprietor or conductor of a drug store or a pharmacy shall be held responsible for the quality of all drugs, chemicals, and medicines he may sell or dispense; and should he knowingly, intentionally, and fraudulently adulterate, or cause to be adulterated, such drugs, chemicals, or medical preparations, he shall be deemed guilty of a misdemeanor, and, upon conviction thereof, be liable to a penalty not exceeding one hundred dollars, and in addition thereto his name stricken from the register.

SEC. 11. Nothing hereinbefore contained in this act shall apply to any practitioner of medicine who does not keep open shop for retailing, dispensing, or compounding of medicines or poisons, nor prevent him from administering or supplying to his patients such articles as he may deem fit and proper. And it is also provided that in rural districts, where there is no registered pharmacist within five miles, it shall be lawful for retail dealers to procure license from the board of pharmacy at a fee of two dollars and fifty cents annually, to sell the usual domestic remedies and medicines, not including any articles enumerated in the schedules A and B of this act.

SEC. 12. Repealed.

SEC. 13. Any person who shall procure, or attempt to procure, registration for himself or for another under this act by making or causing to be made any false representation, and any registered pharmacist who shall be in the habit of being intoxicated, shall be deemed guilty of a misdemeanor, and shall, upon conviction thereof, be liable to a penalty of not less than twenty-five nor more than one hundred dollars; and the name of the person so fraudulently registered shall be stricken from the register.

SEC. 14. This act shall take effect and be in force from and after its publication in the statutes.

Approved March 5, 1885.

## CHAPTER 174.

AN ACT amendatory of and supplemental to chapter 150 of the session laws of 1885, being an act to prevent incompetent or unauthorized persons from engaging in the practice of pharmacy; also to regulate the sale of poisons and proprietary medicines; to prevent and punish the adulteration of drugs, medicines, medical preparations, and chemicals, and to create a board of pharmacy in the State of Kansas and repeal the original sections 2, 4, 5, 6, 9, and 12 of said chapter.

*Be it enacted by the Legislature of the State of Kansas:*

SECTION 1. That section 2 of chapter 150 of the session laws of 1885, be, and the same is hereby, amended so as to read as follows: Section 2. Immediately upon the passage of this act the governor shall appoint five reputable and practicing pharmacists, doing business in the State of Kansas. Said pharmacists, so appointed, shall constitute the board of pharmacy of the State of Kansas and shall hold office as respectively designated in their appointments—two for the term of one year, two for the term of two years, and one for the term of three years respectively, as hereinafter provided, and until their successors have been duly appointed and qualified. The Kansas State pharmaceutical association shall annually nominate and certify to the governor the names of ten registered pharmacists, residents of the State of Kansas, and who are at that time actually engaged in the business of pharmacy and have had ten years' practical experience in dispensing physicians' prescriptions, from which list the governor shall annually appoint one or more pharmacists to fill the vacancy annually occurring in said board. The term of office in said board shall be three years. In case of death, resignation, or removal from State of any member of the said board, or from a vacancy occurring from any cause, the governor shall fill the vacancy by appointing a registered pharmacist from the list last certified to him to serve as a member of the board for the remainder of the term. It shall be the duty of the members of this board, after the receipt of notification of their appointment, to make and subscribe to an oath properly and faithfully to discharge the duties of their office, and within thirty days thereafter meet and organize by the election of a president, secretary, and treasurer, to be selected from the members of the board.

SEC. 2. That section 5 of the act of 1885, to which this act is amendatory, shall read as follows: Section 5. Any person desiring to become a registered pharmacist under the provisions of this act shall, within ninety days after this act shall take effect, forward to said board his affidavit, properly sworn to before the clerk of the district court of the county where such person proposes to engage in the business, showing that such applicant was at the time of the taking effect of this act and ever since has been engaged in the business of preparing and dispensing medicines and physicians' prescriptions within the State of Kansas, and that he has had five years' experience in such business, two years of which experience shall have been in the State of Kansas as a clerk or proprietor, and such affidavit shall be accompanied with the clerk's certificate, showing that he is acquainted with the applicant and knows him to be a person of good moral character and worthy of belief. And such applicant shall, in addition to such affidavit and certificate, present to said board the affidavit of two creditable witnesses substantiating in each material particular the affidavit of such applicant, and, in addition thereto, showing that such applicant is not in the habit of using intoxicants as a beverage, which affidavit shall show the age, residence, and occupation of such witnesses. The board of pharmacy, if satisfied with such proof, shall, upon the presentation of such proof and upon receipt of a fee of $2, register such applicant as a registered pharmacist, and shall thereupon issue to such applicant a certificate of registration, which certificate shall constantly be exposed conspicuously in the pharmacy to which it applies. Persons not availing themselves of the provisions of this section within the time specified may appear before said board for examination as provided by law. The board may register as registered pharmacists, without examination, graduates of recognized schools of pharmacy: *Provided*, Said board shall be satisfied with the moral fitness and sobriety of such graduate: *And provided, further*, That all persons holding certificates by examination as registered pharmacists, issued within two years prior to the taking effect of this act, shall be entitled to registration under this act, and at the end of sixty days after the taking effect of this act any certificate issued before this act took effect shall be no longer of any validity.

SEC. 3. That section 9, of the act of which this is amendatory, shall be, and the same is hereby, amended so as to read as follows: Section 9. Said board of pharmacy shall meet at least once in three months, in at least four different parts of the State in each year, to perform the duties required by this act. The members of the board shall receive the sum of three dollars for each day engaged, together with actual traveling expenses, in the performance of the duties required of them by law, except the secretary who shall receive the sum of six hundred dollars per year, together with all necessary traveling expenses, all to be paid from the treasury of the Kansas board of pharmacy. All fees collected under the provisions of this act shall be paid over at once to the treasurer of said board, and there to be held in trust for the payment of the expenses of said board. And the treasurer of said board shall give such bond from time to time as the board may direct.

SEC. 4. That section 12 of said act, to which this is amendatory, be, and the same is hereby, amended so as to read as follows: Section 12. Pharmacists registered as herein provided shall have the right to keep and sell under such restrictions as herein provided, all medicines and poisons authorized by the National, American, or United

States dispensatory pharmacopœia as of recognized medicinal utility: *Provided*, That nothing herein contained shall be construed so as to shield any apothecary or pharmacist who violates or in anywise abuses this trust for the legitimate and actual necessities of medicines, from the utmost rigor of the law relating to the sale of intoxicating liquors; and upon conviction of any violation of the prohibitory liquor law, his name shall be stricken from the register. It shall be unlawful for any person, on and after the passage of this act, to retail any articles enumerated in schedules A, B, C, except as follows:

### SCHEDULE A.

Arsenic and its preparations, corrosive sublimate, white precipitate, red precipitate, biniodide of mercury, cyanide of potassium, hydro-cyanic acid, chloroform, strychnine, morphine, and all other poisonous vegetable alkaloids and their salts, essential oil of bitter almonds, opium and its preparations, except paregoric and other preparations of opium containing less than two grains to the ounce.

### SCHEDULE B.

Aconite, belladonna, colchicum, conium, nux vomica, henbane, cantharides, creosote, digitalis, and their pharmaceutical preparations; croton oil, chloral hydrate, sulphate of zinc, sugar of lead, mineral acids, carbolic acid, oxalic acid, and all other virulent poisons.

### SCHEDULE C.

Oil of savin, oil of tansy, ergot and its preparations, cotton root and its preparations, and all other active emenagogues or abortives. Articles enumerated in schedules A and B shall not be sold without distinctly labeling the box, vessel, or paper in which the said poison is contained, and also the outside wrapper or cover, with the name of the article, the word "poison," and the name and place of business of the seller. Nor shall it be lawful for any person to sell or deliver any poison enumerated in schedules A and B, unless upon due inquiry it be found that the purchaser is aware of its poisonous character and represents that it is to be used for a legitimate purpose; nor shall it be lawful for any proprietor or owner of any drug store or pharmacy, or any registered pharmacist, to sell or deliver any articles included in the schedules A and B without, before delivering the same to the purchaser, causing an entry to be made in a book kept for that purpose, stating the date of sale, the article sold, the quantity thereof, the purpose for which it is represented by the purchaser to be required, the name of the dispenser, and the name and address of the purchaser, signed by himself; such book to be always open for inspection by the proper authorities, and to be preserved for at least five years. No articles enumerated in schedule C shall be sold except on the prescription of a legally qualified physician. The provisions of this section shall not apply to the sales of poisons to practicing physicians and photographers, and to the dispensing of poison in not unusual doses or quantities upon the prescriptions of licensed practitioners of medicine. All prescriptions of practicing physicians shall be retained by the dispenser. Any person procuring from any pharmacist articles enumerated in schedule A, B, and C, under fraudulent representations, shall be deemed guilty of a misdemeanor, and be liable to a fine of not less than twenty-five nor more than one hundred dollars.

SEC. 5. Any person who may desire a certificate as registered assistant pharmacist, shall apply to the board of pharmacy for examination, and shall pay to the secretary of said board the sum of three dollars, if the board find that he has had two years' experience in a drug store or pharmacy, where physicians' prescriptions were compounded and dispensed, and is otherwise duly qualified they shall duly register him and issue him a certificate as registered assistant pharmacist. In case of a failure to pass a satisfactory examination, a second examination shall be granted him at any meeting of the board within six months, without further payment. No registered assistant pharmacist shall open or conduct a pharmacy on his own account, or be granted a certificate as registered pharmacist until he has passed an examination as herein provided.

SEC. 6. Nothing in this act or of the acts of which this is supplemental and amendatory shall be so construed as to prohibit the employment in any pharmacy of an apprentice for the purpose of being instructed in the practice of pharmacy, but such apprentice shall not be permitted to prepare and dispense physicians' prescriptions, or to sell or furnish poisons, except in the presence and under the supervision of a registered pharmacist or a registered assistant pharmacist.

SEC. 7. It shall be the duty of the State board of pharmacy to investigate all complaints of disregard, noncompliance with or violations of the provisions of this act, and the act to which this is supplemental and amendatory, and to bring all such cases to the notice of the county attorney of the county where such person is doing business, and it shall be the duty of such county attorney to diligently prosecute to effect any such violation.

SEC. 8. Said State board of pharmacy shall, on or before the 10th day of January of each year, make annual report to the governor of its proceedings for the preceding calendar year, together with an account of all moneys received and disbursed by them in pursuance of this act.

SEC. 9. The secretary of the State board of pharmacy shall, on the application of any party, issue to such applicant a certificate or statement showing that the person named in the application is a registered pharmacist, a registered assistant pharmacist, or either, as the case may be. The secretary shall be entitled to and receive a fee of twenty-five cents for each such certificate or statement which he may issue, such fee to accompany the application.

SEC. 10. Original sections two, four, five, six, nine, and twelve of chapter one hundred and fifty of the session laws of 1885 are hereby repealed.

SEC. 11. This act shall take effect and be in force from and after its publication in the official State paper.

## KENTUCKY.

### CHAPTER 492.

AN ACT to establish a State board of pharmacy, defining its duties and powers, and to regulate the practice of pharmacy in the Commonwealth of Kentucky.

*Be it enacted by the General Assembly of the Commonwealth of Kentucky:*

SECTION 1. That within sixty days after the passage of this act the governor shall appoint five persons from among the pharmacists of the State, who have been recommended by the Kentucky pharmaceutical association, which recommendation shall include not less than ten of said pharmacists, who shall constitute the Kentucky board of pharmacy. It shall be the duty of each member of said board, before entering upon the discharge of his duties, to appear before an officer authorized to administer oaths in this State, and make oath to properly and faithfully discharge the duties of a member of the board.

SEC. 2. One of the said members shall hold office for one year, one for two years, one for three years, one for four years, and one for five years, which term shall be determined by vote at the first meeting of said board of pharmacy. The members of the board shall meet at such time and place as may be designated by the member whose name is first on the list of appointments, and shall first proceed to determine by vote the respective terms for which they shall serve, and shall organize by electing a president, treasurer, and secretary, who shall hold their offices for the term of one year, or until their successors are elected and qualified. They shall receive such compensation as the board may fix. Thereafter the board shall meet at least twice in each year, and any three members of the board shall constitute a quorum. The board shall have power to make such by-laws as it may deem necessary, not inconsistent with the constitution of this State or with the provisions of this act.

SEC. 3. The Kentucky pharmaceutical association shall, at each annual meeting, nominate four (4) registered pharmacists, from whom the governor shall fill the vacancy annually occurring in said board, and the person so appointed shall qualify, as provided in section 1, and hold his office for five years. In case of a vacancy occurring in the board from any other cause than expiration of time, the governor shall fill the vacancy by appointment from the list of nominations last made. Removal from the State or permanent discontinuance of business shall be considered a vacation of this office.

SEC. 4. It shall be the duty of said board to examine all applications for registration submitted in proper form, to grant certificates of registration to such persons as may be entitled to the same under the provisions of this act; to report annually to the governor, and to the Kentucky State pharmaceutical association, upon the condition of Pharmacy in the State, which report shall furnish a record of the proceedings of said board for the year and also the names and residences of the pharmacists duly registered under this act.

SEC. 5. The following classes of persons shall be entitled to registration as pharmacists, upon the terms and conditions hereinafter expressed:

*First.* Any person who, at the time of the passage of this act, is carrying on the business of pharmacist on his own account, that is, retailing drugs, medicines, and poisons, and dispensing and compounding prescriptions of medical practitioners, and who shall within six months after the passage of this act forward to said board of pharmacy his affidavit, accompanied by the affidavit of two disinterested persons who are certified, by a county judge or justice of the peace of this State to be reputable citizens, that the applicant was so engaged in business on his own account in this State at the time of the passage of this act.

*Second.* Any person who, at the time of his application, shall have had three years' experience as pharmacist, and who shall pass a satisfactory examination before the State board of pharmacy.

*Third.* Any person who, at the time of the passage of this act, holds a certificate of registration as assistant pharmacist; or who has, for three consecutive years immediately preceding the passage of this act, been engaged as clerk in a retail drug store where prescriptions are compounded, may, with the consent of the board of pharmacy, and without examination, be registered as a pharmacist, and receive a Certificate thereof.

*Fourth.* Graduates of any school or college of pharmacy duly incorporated by the general assembly of Kentucky, which shall, in addition to a theoretical course of study, require at least three years' practical experience in the drug business as a requisite for graduation.

*Fifth.* Any graduate of a regularly incorporated school of medicine who is practicing and compounding medicines in this State, and who, at the time of the passage of this act, had been practicing and compounding medicines in this State for five years immediately preceding the passage of this act.

*Sixth.* Any regular practitioner of medicine who is practicing and compounding medicines in this State, and who, at the time of the passage of this act, had been practicing and compounding medicines in this State for ten years immediately preceding the passage of this act. No person under eighteen years of age shall be entitled to registration under this act as a pharmacist.

SEC. 6. Every applicant for registration under this act shall make written application to the said board of pharmacy for such registration, accompanied by a written statement signed by the applicant in his own hand, and duly verified before an officer authorized to administer oaths in this State, fully setting forth the grounds upon which such application is made. The board of pharmacy shall have power to make such rules and regulations for the examination of applicants for registration, and the granting of certificates and the payment of license fees, as it may see proper, not inconsistent with the provisions of this act: *Provided,* That in cities and towns where the population is five thousand and over, the fee shall not exceed six dollars, and where the population is from three thousand to five thousand, it shall not exceed four dollars, and all under three thousand, shall not exceed two dollars.

SEC. 7. Every application for registration shall be accompanied by the fee fixed by the board. The fee fixed by the board shall, as far as necessary, be devoted to defraying the expenses of the board and paying its officers such compensation as the board may fix.

SEC. 8. It shall be unlawful for any person to retail, compound, or dispense medicines or poisons for medical uses within this State, without first obtaining a certificate of registration as pharmacist from the State board of pharmacy, and causing the same to be recorded in the office of the clerk of the county court in the county wherein said person proposes to carry on such business.

SEC. 9. Before any person who may have registered as a pharmacist, and obtained a certificate thereof, shall commence or continue the business of a pharmacist in any county of this Commonwealth, he shall lodge said certificate with the county clerk of the county wherein such business is carried on or is to be carried on, which shall be recorded by said clerk in a book to be kept in his office for such purpose, and indorse his certificate of such recording on the said certificate of registration, and deliver the same to the owner thereof, within the first ten days of the next ensuing January, and annually thereafter the said pharmacist, if he continue in business or intends to continue in business, shall go before the county court in the county in which he is doing business or intends to do business, and apply for a renewal of his license, and upon producing his certificate of registration he shall be entitled to a renewal certificate, under which he may conduct such business. For each record of certificate of registration the county clerk shall be entitled to a fee of fifty cents, which shall be paid by the pharmacist receiving same. It shall be the duty of each county court clerk in this State to keep constantly at hand a correct list of the registered pharmacists in the county whose certificates are recorded in his office, and of the renewals issued by him, and report same in writing to every grand jury impaneled at the regular term of the circuit court in his county, and during the month of February of each year he shall make a full and correct list of the registered pharmacists in his county and forward the same to the secretary of the State board of pharmacy. For each failure to perform his duties under this act such clerk shall, upon conviction, be fined fifty dollars by warrant, in any court having jurisdiction thereof.

SEC. 10. Any person not being a registered pharmacist, or who shall not have complied with all the provisions of this act, who shall take, exhibit, or use the title of pharmacist, or who proposes to or does compound or dispense prescriptions of medical practitioners, or retail medicines or poisons to be used as medicines, or shall in any way violate the provisions of this act, shall be subject to indictment for each offense, and upon conviction shall be fined, for the first offense, twenty-five dollars and the cost of prosecution, and upon indictment and conviction for a second offense under this act shall be fined fifty dollars and the cost of prosecution, and for each subsequent violation he shall be fined one hundred dollars and the cost of prosecution.

SEC. 11. All prosecutions under this act shall be in the name of the Commonwealth of Kentucky, and all fines imposed and collected under such prosecutions, after payment of all costs and expenses of such prosecutions, including the usual commission to the prosecuting attorney, shall be paid over to the trustee of the jury fund in the county where such fines are imposed, and by him reported and paid to the auditor of public accounts for the State, as other public moneys collected by him are by law required to be reported and paid over. And all such sums thus reported and paid over shall go into and become a part of the common fund of the State.

SEC. 12. Nothing in this act shall be construed to apply to the business of a licensed practitioner of medicine, nor to prevent such practitioner from supplying his patients with such articles as he may deem proper; but no licensed practitioner of medicine shall be entitled to carry on or conduct the practice or business of pharmacy in this State without obtaining registration as a pharmacist; nor to those who sell medicines or poisons by wholesale only; nor to the manufacture or sale of proprietary medicines. Nothing in this act shall be so construed as to prohibit the employment in any pharmacy of apprentices or assistants for the purpose of being instructed in the practice of pharmacy; but such apprentices or assistants shall not be permitted to prepare or dispense physicians' prescriptions, or to sell or furnish medicines or poisons, except in the presence of and under the personal supervision of a pharmacist registered and licensed under this act; nor to prevent any one not a registered pharmacist under this act from owning a pharmacy, provided the duties and business of pharmacy are in charge of and under the control of a registered pharmacist under this act.

SEC. 13. Nothing in this act will be so construed so as to prohibit any person from selling the following articles, to wit: Cream of tartar, spirits of camphor, soda, tincture of iron, sal soda, castor oil, salts, calomel, Paris green, sweet oil, blue stone, ipecac, acids, spirits of turpentine, peruvian bark, and all its salts and preparations; aqua ammonia, essence of peppermint, spirits of nitro, essence of cinnamon, carbonate iron, copperas, tincture of iron, borax, glycerine, sulphur, paregoric, essence of ginger, syrup of ipecac, and syrup squills.

SEC. 14. Persons who at the time of the passage of this act hold certificates of registration as pharmacists or assistant pharmacists shall not be required to register under this act, but shall file their certificates of registration with the county clerk for record and take out renewals thereof, as provided in section 2 of this act, and in all other respects shall be amenable to the provisions of this act.

SEC. 15. Nothing in this act shall be so construed as to apply to towns or cities of less than one thousand inhabitants.

SEC. 16. An act entitled "An act to regulate the sale of medicines and poisons," approved February twenty-first, eighteen hundred and seventy-four, and an act amendatory thereto, approved March eighteenth, eighteen hundred and seventy-six; and all acts or parts of acts, whether general or special or private, in conflict with this act are hereby repealed.

SEC. 17. This act shall take effect from and after its passage.

Approved March 13, 1888.

By the governor,

S. B. BUCKNER.

GEO. M. ADAMS,
*Secretary of State.*

BEN. JOHNSON,
*Speaker of the House of Representatives.*
J. W. BRYAN,
*Speaker of the Senate.*

## LOUISIANA.

AN ACT to regulate the practice of pharmacy; to regulate the sale of compounded medicines and drugs, preparations and prescriptions; to regulate the sale of poisons; to create a State board of pharmacy, and to regulate the fees and emoluments thereof; to prevent the practice of pharmacy by unauthorized persons; and to provide for the trial and punishment of violators of the provisions of this act by fine or imprisonment.

SECTION 1. *Be it enacted by the General Assembly of the State of Louisiana,* That it shall hereafter be unlawful for any other than a registered pharmacist to compound medicines, drugs or chemicals, or to institute or conduct any apothecary or drug store, or pharmacy shop for compounding drugs, medicines, or chemicals, or for any person to be employed therein, or placed in charge thereof, for the purpose of compounding drugs or chemicals under prescriptions or otherwise.

SEC. 2. *Be it further enacted, etc.,* Any person twenty-one years of age shall be entitled to registration as a duly registered pharmacist on exhibiting to the board of pharmacy a diploma from any college or school of pharmacy, in Europe or America, of good and respectable standing, the status of the institution as to respectability and standing to be judged and approved by said board, together with the affidavit of the applicant, stating his age, nativity, and that he is the bona fide holder of the diploma and the person named therein, and that he is a regular graduate or alumnus of said institution, or in case that said applicant shall produce no diploma as hereinabove set forth, it shall be sufficient for him to present an affidavit that he has had four years' practical experience in the manipulation and compounding of physicians' prescriptions under the supervision of a registered pharmacist, who shall also attest the truth of the said affidavit by swearing thereto, if said registered pharmacist be alive and resident in the State of Louisiana; and said affidavit shall set forth the age of the applicant, the place of his nativity, and when and where he has practiced pharmacy, said affidavits to be preserved on the file by the board of pharmacy as a part of its records.

SEC. 3. *Be it further enacted, etc.*, That the foregoing provisions of this act shall not apply to or effect any person who shall be engaged in the actual preparation, compounding, and dispensing of medicines or drugs in the drug and apothecary business as proprietor of the same, or as qualified assistant therein at the time of the passage of this act, except in so far as relates to registration and fees provided in section five. A qualified assistant engaged in the business at the time of the passage of this act is one who has had not less than two years' practical experience in the preparation, compounding, and dispensing of medicines or drugs in the drug and apothecary business. All other actual assistants actually engaged in the business at the time of the passage of this act shall, upon the completion of a like term of two years' experience, be entitled to registration as qualified assistants without examination: *Provided*, That nothing contained in this act shall in any manner whatever interfere with the business of any registered practitioner of medicine, nor in any way prevent him from administering or supplying his patients with such drugs and medicines as he may deem fit and proper, nor shall it interfere with the making and dealing in proprietary remedies, popularly called patent medicines, nor prevent storekeepers from dealing in and selling the commonly used standard medicines and poisons, if all such standard medicines and poison included in this section conform in all respects to the requirements of section seven. Nor shall this act apply to any planter furnishing medicines to hands in his employment or leasing lands from him.

SEC. 4. *Be it further enacted, etc.*, That in case the board of pharmacy shall have reason to doubt the truth of the allegations of any affidavit made under the provisions of the foregoing section, it shall have the right to examine into and hear evidence thereon, and if convinced of the falsity thereof it shall have the right to refuse registration, subject to the right of the applicant to appeal to the courts by mandamus: *Provided*, That false swearing in an affidavit hereinbefore mentioned shall be deemed perjury, and liable to punishment as in other cases under existing laws.

SEC. 5. *Be it further enacted, etc.*, That where the applicant neither furnishes the diploma or affidavit required by the foregoing sections, he shall have the right to registration after having passed a satisfactory examination by the board of pharmacy as to his qualifications and capacity, which board shall thereupon register the applicant, and shall grant to him a certificate of registration as a pharmacist, the same as in the case of the production of a diploma or affidavit as hereinbefore provided. The board of pharmacy may grant certificates of registration to licentiates of such other State boards, or the duly constituted authorities of other countries, without further examination. The board of pharmacy shall have the right to exact and collect from applicants, before issuance of a certificate, five dollars ($5) for an examination of the applicant and three dollars ($3) for the issuance of the certificate.

SEC. 6. *Be it further enacted, etc.*, That the governor shall appoint the board of pharmacy, consisting of nine (9) reputable practicing pharmacists doing business in the State, who shall serve for four (4) years from date of their appointment; any vacancy shall be filled for the unexpired term by the governor's appointment. Said board shall elect a president and an officer to be known as the secretary and treasurer, and in addition to its duties in holding examinations and granting certificates it shall report to the prosecuting officer of the State of Louisiana all persons violating the provisions of this act; it shall report annually to the governor of the State upon the condition of pharmacy in the State, any recommendations for the improvement of its practice, as well as a record of the proceedings of the board during the year, and the names of all pharmacists duly registered under this act; and the fees collected under the provisions of this act shall be applied to the payment of the expenses of the board in such manner as it shall direct.

SEC. 7. *Be it further enacted, etc.*, That all pharmacists, druggists, or apothecaries shall label all bottles, vials, jars, boxes, parcels, packages, or other receptacles or coverings, or wrappings of drugs, medicines, or chemicals sold or dispensed by them, with a label in legible writing or printed letters giving the name of the proprietor of the store, the name of the physician prescribing, or shop and the place of sale of said drug, medicine, or chemical; and in case the medicine, drug, or chemical be of a nature poisonous to the human system or to animals said label shall have printed thereon a skull and crossbones, with the word "Poison" in large, heavy lettering. All prescriptions shall have in addition thereto a number, the name of the person actually and personally compounding the same, the directions for its use internally or externally, and the date of its compounding.

SEC. 8. *Be it further enacted, etc.*, That any person offending against any provisions of this act shall be deemed guilty of a misdemeanor against the State of Louisiana, and shall be prosecuted before any court of criminal jurisdiction, and if adjudged guilty shall pay a fine of not less than fifty dollars ($50) nor more than one hundred dollars ($100), and in default of payment thereof shall be imprisoned in the parish jail for not more than thirty (30) days.

SEC. 9. *Be it further enacted, etc.*, That this act shall take effect thirty (30) days after its promulgation.

S. P. HENRY,<br>
*Speaker of the House of Representatives.*<br>
JAMES JEFFRIES,<br>
*Lieutenant-Governor and President of the Senate.*

Approved, July 11, 1888.

FRANCIS T. NICHOLLS,<br>
*Governor of the State of Louisiana.*

OPINION OF HON. WALTER H. ROGERS, ATTORNEY-GENERAL OF THE STATE OF LOUISIANA.

Act 66 of 1888 does not repeal but modifies section 2, act 70 of 1877, in so far as to fix the qualifications and determine who, under the law, is a licensed druggist.

Act 27 of 1879, section 16, is a revenue act fixing the amount of license to be paid as a privilege in pursuing the occupation. The proviso as to qualification is controlled by act 66 of 1888.

If a regular practitioner of medicine also engages in the practice of pharmacy, institutes or conducts any apothecary or drug store or pharmacy shop, he comes under the provision of act 66, the exception as to him being simply as to furnishing or administering drugs to his patients, the law evidently having in contemplation the "saddle bags" of the doctor, and not a permanent establishment, as defined in section 1 of act 66 of 1888.

EXTRACT FROM ACT 70 OF 1877, LAWS OF LOUISIANA.

SEC. 2. *Be it enacted*, That merchants, where there is no licensed drug store within eight miles of the place where such merchant is doing business, selling drugs in original packages, prepared and labeled by any licensed druggist, shall not be required to pay druggists' license.

# MAINE.

## CHAPTER 379.

AN ACT To prevent incompetent persons from conducting the business of apothecaries.

*Be it enacted by the Senate and House of Representatives in Legislature assembled, as follows:*

SECTION 1. From and after the passage of this act it shall not be lawful for any person, within the limits of the State, to conduct the business of an apothecary, or any part thereof, except as hereinafter provided.

SEC. 2. The governor, under the advice and consent of the council, shall appoint three suitable persons to be commissioners of pharmacy, one commissioner to be appointed as the term of each of those now holding office shall expire, to hold office for the term of three years, unless removed for cause, and until a successor is appointed and qualified. If a vacancy occurs in said commission another shall be appointed as aforesaid to fill the unexpired term thereof. Before entering on the duties of their office the commissioners shall be sworn to faithfully and impartially discharge the same, and a record shall be made thereof on their commission. Said commissioners shall make a report of their proceedings annually to the governor and council, who shall cause such a number of said reports to be printed as they deem necessary.

SEC. 3. Said commissioners shall examine any person who desires to carry on the business of an apothecary, and if he is found skilled in pharmacy, shall give him a certificate of that fact and that he is authorized to engage in the business of an apothecary, and such certificate must be signed by at least two commissioners. They shall register in a suitable book, to be kept in the office of the secretary of state, the name and place of residence of all to whom they issue certificates, and the date thereof.

SEC. 4. Every person not now registered, unless he was engaged in the business of apothecary in the State of Maine, on the eleventh day of March, in the year of our Lord eighteen hundred and seventy-seven, continuing in or hereafter entering on the business of an apothecary, shall be examined by said commissioners, and shall present to them satisfactory evidence that he has been an apprentice, or employed in an apothecary store where physicians' prescriptions are compounded, at least three years; or has graduated from some regularly incorporated medical college or college of pharmacy, and is competent for the business; and the commissioners may then grant him a certificate and registry as hereinbefore provided; but only one of the partners in a firm need be a registered druggist, provided the partner who compounds medicines be registered. And any physician who has a diploma as a graduate of a duly established medical college in the United States, and in active practice, may do the business of an apothecary without being registered.

SEC. 5. For each examination under the provisions of this act, the commissioners shall be entitled to receive from the person examined ten dollars, except as hereinafter provided, which shall be in full for all services and expenses. In case the result of the examination is unsatisfactory, and no certificate is granted, the applicant shall have the right to another examination without charge after an interval of two months and within twelve months after the date of his first examination.

SEC. 6. Certificates of two grades or kinds may be issued, whereof one shall declare that the holder is skilled in pharmacy, as in section four of this act, and the other kind, which after the examination of the applicants therefor, may be issued to such as shall be not less than eighteen years of age and who have served two full years in an apothecary store where physicians' prescriptions are compounded, shall declare that the holder is a qualified assistant and is competent to take charge of the business of an apothecary, during the temporary absence of the registered apothecary, and the fee for such assistant's examination shall be five dollars.

SEC. 7. It shall not be lawful for any apothecary store to be kept open for the sale of medicines or poisons, or for compounding physicians' prescriptions, nor shall such drugs or medicines be exposed or displayed for sale in any such store, unless the same is placed and kept under the personal control and supervision of a registered apothecary or qualified assistant, but such store may be under the charge of a qualified assistant during the temporary absence of such registered apothecary.

SEC. 8. Any person engaged in the business of apothecary in the State of Maine on the eleventh day of March, in the year of our Lord one thousand eight hundred and seventy-seven, may receive a certificate and be registered as aforesaid on application to said commissioners with proof of his competency.

SEC. 9. If any person who was not engaged in the business of an apothecary within the State of Maine on the eleventh day of March, in the year of our Lord one thousand eight hundred and seventy-seven, shall hereafter engage in or be found in charge of or carrying on the business of an apothecary contrary to provisions of this act, he shall upon indictment and conviction be subject to a penalty of fifty dollars per month for the first offense, and one hundred dollars per month for each and every subsequent offense whether for continuance in said business or for engaging anew therein in violation of the provisions of this act. It is hereby made the duty of the county attorney in each county, upon complaint made by any one of said commissioners, to prosecute all violations of the provisions of this act. The treasurer of each county shall pay to the treasurer of the law library association of his county for the use and benefit of the county law library, twenty per cent of all fines actually paid into the county treasury for the violation of any of the provisions of this act.

SEC. 10. The provisions of this act shall apply in the cases of women who shall hereafter enter upon and carry on the business of apothecaries.

SEC. 11. This act shall not apply in the case of physicians who prepare and dispense their own medicines, nor to the sale of proprietary preparations.

SEC. 12. All acts and parts of acts inconsistent with this act are hereby repealed.

SEC. 13. Any person may enter upon the business of an apothecary without the certificate required by the foregoing act, provided he does not personally do the duties of an apothecary, but employs a duly registered apothecary who has sole charge of compounding, putting up, and dispensing medicines and drugs under the provisions of this act.

SEC. 14. No action now pending by virtue of section six of chapter twenty-eight of the revised statutes shall be maintained except as to costs, or shall hereafter be commenced for any penalty or forfeiture incurred prior to the approval of this act.

SEC. 15. The word apothecary as used in this act shall not include persons who do not compound medicines, put up prescriptions, or sell poisons.

SEC. 16. This act shall take effect when approved.

[As amended by act approved March 25, 1893.]

## MARYLAND.

AN ACT to repeal sections 388 to 396, inclusive, of article IV of the public local laws, title "City of Baltimore," subtitle "Commissioners of pharmacy and practical chemistry," and to reënact the same with amendments.

SECTION 1. Be it enacted by the General Assembly of Maryland, that sections 388, 389, 390, 391, 392, 393, 394, 395, and 396, inclusive, of article IV of public local laws, title "City of Baltimore," subtitle "Commissioners of pharmacy and practical chemistry," be, and the same are hereby, repealed and reënacted with amendments so as to read as follows:

SEC. 388. That the term or name pharmacist in the meaning and scope of this act does mean, embrace, and apply to all persons engaged in vending, at retail, drugs, medicines, and chemicals for medicinal use, and in compounding and dispensing physicians' prescriptions, either as owner of stores, as managing assistants, or as relief clerks in temporary charge of stores.

SEC. 389. That any person who, after the passage of this act, does or shall vend, at retail, poisonous drugs for medicinal use, or compound or dispense physicians' prescriptions in the city of Baltimore without complying with the requirements of this act, shall be deemed guilty of a misdemeanor, and be subject to a penalty or fine of fifty dollars ($50) for each and every week he shall continue to vend, at retail, poisonous drugs for medicinal use, or compound or dispense physicians' prescriptions in violation of this act; said penalty or fine to be sued for in the name of the State of Maryland before a justice of the peace, as small debts are now recoverable; said penalty or fine to go to the Maryland board of pharmacy, appointed under this act, to be used as a fund for carrying out the provisions of this act; and it shall be the duty of the State's attorney of the city of Baltimore, at the request of said board of pharmacy, to prosecute any person who shall have violated any requirement of this act: *Provided*, That nothing in this act shall be so construed as to prevent any practicing physician from supplying medicines in connection with professional practice, nor to restrict the sale, at retail, of patent and proprietary medicines and compounds prepared and compounded for medical use by wholesale dealers in drugs and medicines, when sold in original package—box or bottle; and no penalty shall hereafter be enforced against any person for the sale of patent or proprietary medicines or compounds prepared by wholesale dealers in drugs and medicines when sold as aforesaid; and no penalty shall hereafter be enforced against any person for the sale of proprietary or patent medicines or drugs other than poisonous.

SEC. 390. That the Maryland College of Pharmacy shall nominate, biennially, of the most skilled and competent pharmacists of the city of Baltimore ten (10) persons, from amongst whom the governor shall appoint three (3) commissioners, whose duty it shall be to faithfully and impartially execute, or cause to be executed, all the provisions and requirements of this act. They shall, upon application and in such manner and in such place as they may determine, examine each and every person who shall desire to engage in vending, at retail, drugs, medicines, or chemicals for medicinal use, or in compounding and dispensing physicians' prescriptions in the city of Baltimore, touching his competency and qualifications, and upon being satisfied that the person so examined is competent and qualified to vend, at retail, drugs, medicines, and chemicals for medicinal use, and compound and dispense physicians' prescriptions safely, and without jeopardy to the health and lives of the people of the city of Baltimore, they or any two of them shall grant such person a certificate of competency and register him as a pharmacist.

SEC. 391. That the commissioners appointed under this act shall be styled and known as the "Commissioners of Pharmacy and Practical Chemistry," and shall hold office for two years and thereafter, until their successors have been appointed and have qualified. Said commissioners shall, within thirty (30) days after notification of their appointment, each subscribe to an oath before the clerk of the superior court of Baltimore city to impartially and faithfully discharge the duties prescribed by this act. The position of any commissioner appointed under this act who shall fail to qualify within the time and in the manner named shall be vacant. The governor shall fill all vacancies occurring from amongst the persons nominated by the Maryland College of Pharmacy under section 390 of this act.

SEC. 392. That each and every person, before commencing to vend, at retail, drugs, medicines, or chemicals for medicinal use, or to compound or dispense physicians' prescriptions in the city of Baltimore, as managing owner of a store, or as managing assistant of a store, or as relief clerk temporarily in charge of a store, shall register as a pharmacist under the provisions of this act. That every person who shall at the time that this act goes into effect be engaged in vending, at retail, drugs, medicines, and chemicals for medicinal use, and compounding and dispensing physicians' prescriptions in the city of Baltimore, and registered as pharmacist under an act entitled "An act to prevent incompetent persons from conducting business as pharmacists, or vending, at retail, drugs, medicines, or chemicals for medicinal use in the city of Baltimore," approved April 1st, 1872, and amended by the repeal and reënactment of sections 2 and 9, chapter 91, passed at January session, 1876, shall be deemed competent to register as a pharmacist within the meaning of this act. That every person holding a diploma from a regular chartered and recognized college or school of pharmacy, based upon a full apprenticeship of four years, as a pharmacist, and who presents satisfactory evidence of these facts to the said commissioners of pharmacy and practical chemistry, shall be deemed competent, and entitled to register as a pharmacist.

SEC. 393. That said commissioners of pharmacy and practical chemistry shall demand and receive from each applicant for registration whom they examine five (5) dollars for each examination, and shall likewise be entitled to demand and receive one (1) dollar from every person whom they register or re-register, which money so received under the provisions of this section shall be used and applied by said board to defray the expenses accruing or arising under this act. And that every pharmacist, managing assistant, and relief clerk in the city of Baltimore shall re-register annually, after his first registration, during the term he shall continue in the practice of his profession, on such date as the board of pharmacy may determine, and shall pay to the said board the fee of one (1) dollar as provided in this section, for which he shall receive a renewal of said registration.

SEC. 394. That in case of the death of a registered pharmacist, doing business as such in the city of Baltimore, his legal representative may continue said business for the benefit of the estate of said deceased under the control and management of a registered pharmacist, subject to all the requirements of this act.

SEC. 395. That no person, unless he be registered as a pharmacist under this act or unless he be an apprentice who has had at least two years' experience under a pharmacist, or who has attended at least one full course of lectures on pharmacy, chemistry and materia medica, shall be permitted to compound and dispense the prescriptions, except under the supervison of a registered pharmacist. Any registered pharmacist violating this section, or permitting its violation in any store under his charge or management, shall be subject to a penalty or fine of not more than fifty (50) dollars, which fines are to be disposed of as provided in section 393.

SEC. 396. That all acts and parts of acts, so far as they may be in conflict with this act, are hereby declared void and of no effect.

SEC. 397. Any person who shall mix with any substance or preparation used, or intended to be used as an officinal medicine, any foreign or inert substance for the purpose of adulterating or weakening the same, or shall knowingly sell or knowingly offer for sale any officinal medicines so adulterated or deficient in standard strength, shall be deemed guilty of a misdemeanor and subject to a penalty or fine of fifty (50) dollars, as provided in the preceding section.

## MONTANA.

Has no pharmacy law.

## MASSACHUSETTS.

[Chapter 313, Acts of 1885.]

AN ACT to establish a board of registration in pharmacy.

*Be it enacted, etc., as follows:*

SECTION 1. The governor of the Commonwealth, with the advice and consent of the council, shall appoint, after the passage of this act, five skilled pharmacists, resident in the Commonwealth, who have had ten consecutive years of practical experience in the compounding and dispensing of physicians' prescriptions, who shall constitute a board of registration in pharmacy. Such persons shall be appointed and hold office, beginning on the first day of October next, one for one year, one for two years, one for three years, one for four years, and one for five years, or until their successors shall be appointed; and the governor shall appoint annually thereafter before the first day of October in each year one skilled pharmacist, qualified as aforesaid, to hold office for five years from the first day of October next ensuing. Not more than one member of said board shall be interested in the sale of drugs, medicines, and chemicals, and the compounding and dispensing of physicians' prescriptions in the same city or town. All vacancies occurring in said board shall be filled in accordance with the provisions of this act for the establishment of the original board. Any member of said board may be removed from office for cause by the governor with the advice and consent of the council.

SEC. 2. The members of said board shall meet on the first Tuesday of October next, at such time and place as they may determine, and shall immediately proceed to organize by electing a president and secretary who shall be members of the board and who shall hold their respective offices for the term of one year. The secretary shall give to the treasurer and receiver-general of the Commonwealth a bond with sufficient sureties, to be approved by the governor and council, for the faithful discharge of the duties of his office. The said board shall hold three regular meetings in each year, one on the first Tuesday of January, one on the first Tuesday of May, and one on the first Tuesday of October, and such additional meetings at such times and places as they may determine.

SEC. 3. Repealed May, 1887; such repeal not to impair or affect the rights or privileges of any person hitherto registered as a pharmacist under the provisions of said section.

SEC. 4. Any person not entitled to registration as aforesaid shall, upon payment of a fee of five dollars, be entitled to examination, and if found qualified shall be registered as a pharmacist, and shall receive the certificate thereof provided for in section three. Any person may be reëxamined at any regular meeting of the board upon the payment of a fee of three dollars. All fees received by the board under this act shall be paid by the secretary of the board into the treasury of the Commonwealth once in each month.

SEC. 5. The compensation, incidental and traveling expenses of the board shall be paid from the treasury of the Commonwealth. The compensation of the board shall be five dollars each for every day actually spent in the discharge of their duties, and three cents per mile each way for necessary traveling expenses in attending the meetings of the board, but in no case shall any more be paid than was actually expended. Such compensation and the incidental and traveling expenses shall be approved by the board and sent to the auditor of the Commonwealth who shall certify to the governor and council the amounts due as in case of all other bills and accounts approved by him under the provisions of law: *Provided*, That the amount so paid shall not exceed the amount received by the treasurer and receiver-general of the Commonwealth from the board in fees as herein specified, and so much of said receipts as may be necessary is hereby appropriated for the compensation and expenses of the board as aforesaid.

SEC. 6. The board shall keep a record of the names of all persons registered hereunder, and a record of all moneys received and disbursed by said board, a duplicate whereof shall always be open to inspection in the office of the secretary of the Commonwealth. Said board shall annually report to the governor, on or before the first day of January in each year, the condition of pharmacy in the State, which report shall contain a full and complete record of all its official acts during the year, and shall also contain a statement of the receipts and disbursements of the board.

SEC. 7. It shall be the duty of the board to investigate all complaints of disregard, noncompliance, or violation of the provisions of this act, and to bring all such cases to the notice of the proper prosecuting officers.

SEC. 8. Every person who has received a certificate of registration from the board shall conspicuously display the same in his place of business.

SEC. 9. Whoever not being registered as aforesaid shall, by himself or his agent or servant, unless such agent or servant is so registered, retail, compound for sale, or dispense for medicinal purposes drugs, medicines, chemicals, or poisons shall be punished by a fine not exceeding fifty dollars. But nothing in this act shall be construed to prohibit the employment of apprentices or assistants under the personal supervision of a registered pharmacist.

SEC. 10. This act shall not apply to physicians putting up their own prescriptions or dispensing medicines to their patients; nor to the sale of drugs, medicines, chemicals, or poisons at wholesale only; nor to the manufacture or sale of patent and proprietary medicines; nor to the sale of nonpoisonous domestic remedies usually sold by grocers or others; nor shall any member of a copartnership be liable to the penalties hereof if any other member of such copartnership is a registered pharmacist: *Provided*, That such nonregistered member shall not retail, compound for sale, or dispense for medicinal purposes drugs, medicines, chemicals, or poisons except under the personal supervision of a registered pharmacist.

SEC. 11. For the purpose of the appointment of said board and of registration of persons by them hereunder this act shall take effect upon its passage, and shall take full effect on the first day of January in the year eighteen hundred and eighty-six.

Approved June 11, 1885.

## MICHIGAN.

AN ACT to regulate the practice of pharmacy in the State of Michigan.

SECTION 1. *The people of the State of Michigan enact*, That the governor, with the advice and consent of the senate, shall, within thirty days after the passage of this act, appoint five persons and annually thereafter one person from among such competent pharmacists in the State as have had ten years' practical experience in dispensing physicians' prescriptions, who shall constitute the Michigan board of pharmacy. The term of office of said five persons shall be so arranged that the term of one shall expire on the thirty-first day of December of each year, and all appointments made thereafter shall be for the term of five years.

SEC. 2. The said board shall, within thirty days after its appointment, meet and organize by election of a president and secretary from its own members, who shall be elected for the term of one year, and shall perform the duties prescribed by the board. It shall be the duty of the board to examine all applications for registration submitted in proper form; to grant certificates of registration to such persons as may be entitled to the same under the provisions of this act; to investigate complaints and to cause the prosecution of all persons violating its provisions; to report annually to the governor, and to the Michigan pharmaceutical association, upon the condition of pharmacy in the State, which said report shall also furnish a record of the proceedings of the said board, for the year, and also the names of all pharmacists duly registered under this act. The board shall hold meetings for the examinations of applicants for registration, and the transaction of such other business as shall pertain to its duties, at least once in four months, said meetings to be held on the first Tuesdays of March, July, and November in each year; shall make by-laws for the proper fulfillment of its duties under this act, and shall keep a book of registration in which shall be entered the names and places of business of all persons registered under this act, which book shall also specify such facts as said persons shall claim to justify their registration. The records of said board, or a copy of any part thereof, certified by the secretary to be a true copy, attested by the seal of the board, shall be accepted as competent evidence in all courts of the State. Three members of said board shall constitute a quorum.

SEC. 3. The secretary of the board and treasurer thereof, if such separate officer be created, shall receive a salary which shall be fixed by the board. They shall also receive the amount of their traveling and other expenses incurred in the performance of their official duties. The other members shall receive the sum of three dollars for each day actually engaged in this service, and all legitimate and necessary expenses incurred in the performance of their official duties. Said salaries, per diem, and expenses shall be paid from the fees received under the provisions of this act. All moneys received in excess of said per diem allowance, and other expenses provided for, shall be paid into the State treasury at the end of each year, and so much thereof as shall be necessary to meet the current expenses of said board shall be subject to the order thereof if, in any year, the receipts of said board shall not be equal to its expenses. The board shall make an annual report and render an account to the board of State auditors, and to the Michigan pharmaceutical association, of all moneys received and disbursed by it pursuant to this act.

SEC. 4. Every person who shall, within three months after this act takes effect, forward the board of pharmacy satisfactory proof, supported by his affidavit, that he was engaged in the business of a dispensing pharmacist on his own account in this State at the time this act takes effect, in the preparation of physicians' prescriptions, or that at such time he had been employed or engaged three years or more as a pharmacist in the compounding of physicians' prescriptions, and was at said time so employed in this State, shall, upon the payment to the board of a fee of two dollars, be granted the certificate of a registered pharmacist: *Provided*, That in case of failure or neglect to register as herein provided, then such person shall, in order to be registered, comply with the requirements provided for registration as a licentiate in pharmacy hereafter described.

SEC. 5. No person other than a licentiate in pharmacy shall be entitled to registration as a pharmacist, except as provided in section four. Licentiates in pharmacy shall be such persons, not less than eighteen years of age, who shall have passed a satisfactory examination touching their competency before the board of pharmacy. Every such person shall, before an examination is granted, furnish satisfactory evidence that he is of temperate habits and pay to the board a fee of three dollars: *Provided*, That in case of failure of any applicant to pass a satisfactory examination, the money shall be held to his credit for a second examination at any time within one year. The said board may grant certificates of registration without further examination to the licentiates of such other boards of pharmacy as it may deem proper upon a payment of a fee of two dollars.

SEC. 6. The said board may grant, under such rules and regulations as it may deem proper, at a fee not exceeding one dollar, the certificate of registered assistant to clerks or assistants in pharmacy not less than eighteen years of age, who at the time this act takes effect shall be engaged in such service in this State, and have been employed or engaged two years or more in the practice of pharmacy, but such certificate shall not entitle the holder to engage in such business on his own account, or to take charge of or act as manager of a pharmacy or drug store.

SEC. 7. Each registered pharmacist, or registered assistant, who desires to continue the practice of his profession shall annually, after the expiration of the first year of his registration, during the time he shall continue in such practice, on such date as the board of pharmacy may determine, pay to the said board a registration fee to be fixed by the board, but which shall not exceed one dollar for a pharmacist, or fifty cents for an assistant, for which he shall receive a renewal of said registration. Every person receiving a certificate under this act shall keep the same conspicuously exposed in his place of business. Every registered pharmacist, or assistant, shall, within ten days after changing his place of business or employment, as designated by his certificate, notify the secretary of the board of his new place of business. If any pharmacist or registered assistant shall fail or neglect to procure his annual registration, or to comply with the other provisions of this section, his right to act as such pharmacist or assistant shall cease at the expiration of ten days from the time notice of such failure to comply with the provisions of this section shall have been mailed to him by the secretary of said board.

SEC. 8. All or any registration obtained through false representations shall be void, and the board of pharmacy may hear complaints and evidence, and may revoke such certificates as it may deem improperly held.

SEC. 9. Any proprietor of a pharmacy who, not being a registered pharmacist, shall, ninety days after this act takes effect, fail or neglect to place in charge of such pharmacy a registered pharmacist, or any such proprietor who shall by himself, or any other person, permit the compounding or dispensing of prescriptions, or the vending of drugs, medicines, or poisons, in his store or place of business, except by or in the presence and under the supervision of a registered pharmacist, or except by a registered assistant; or any person not being a registered pharmacist who shall take charge of or act as manager of such pharmacy or store, or who, not being a registered pharmacist or registered assistant, shall retail, compound, or dispense drugs, medicines, or poisons, or any person violating any other provision of this act to which no other penalty is herein attached, shall be deemed guilty of a misdemeanor, and for every such offense, upon conviction thereof, shall be punished by a fine of not less than ten nor more than one hundred dollars, and in default of payment thereof shall be imprisoned not less than ten days nor more than ninety days, or both such fine and imprisonment, in the discretion of the court.

SEC. 10. Nothing in this act shall apply to, or in any manner interfere with, the business of any practicing physician who does not keep open shop for retailing, dispensing, or compounding of medicine and poison, or prevent him from supplying to his patient such articles as may seem to him proper, nor with the vending of patent or proprietary medicines by any retail dealer *who has been in such business three years or more*, nor with the selling by any person of drugs, medicines, chemicals, essential oils, and tinctures which are put up in bottles, boxes, packages, bearing labels securely affixed, which labels shall bear the name of the pharmacist or druggist putting up the same, the dose that may be administered to persons three months, six months, one year, three years, five years, ten years, fifteen years, and twenty-one years of age, and, if a poison, the name or names of the most common antidotes; of copperas, borax, blue vitriol, saltpeter, pepper, sulphur, brimstone, Paris green, licorice, sage, senna leaves, castor oil, sweet oil, spirits of turpentine, glycerin, Glauber salts, Epsom salts, cream tartar, bicarbonate of soda, sugar of lead, and such acids as are used in coloring and tanning, nor with the selling of paregoric, essence of peppermint, essence of ginger, essence of cinnamon, hive syrup, syrup of ipecac, tincture of arnica, syrup of tolu, syrup of squills, spirits of camphor, number six, sweet spirits of nitre, laudanum, quinine, and all other preparations of cinchona bark, tincture of aconite, and tincture of iron, compound cathartic pills, or quinine pills, nor with the exclusively wholesale business of any dealer: *Provided,* That every person who shall, within three months after this act takes effect, forward to the board of pharmacy satisfactory proof, supported by his affidavit, that he was engaged in the business of a dispensing pharmacist on his own account in this State, in the preparation of physicians' prescriptions, three years next previous to the second day of June, 1885, or that at such time he had been employed or engaged three years or more as a pharmacist in the compounding of physicians' prescriptions, and was at said time so employed in this State, shall, upon the payment to the board of a fee of two dollars, be granted the certificate of a registered pharmacist: *And provided, further,* That the said board may grant, at a fee not exceeding one dollar, to such person not less than sixteen years of age who shall pass a satisfactory examination touching his competency before the board of pharmacy the certificate of registered "assistant," but such certificate shall not entitle the holder to engage in business on his own account or to take charge of or act as manager of a pharmacy or drug store.

SEC. 11. No person shall add to or remove from any drug, medicine, chemical, pharmaceutical preparation any ingredient or material for the purpose of adulteration or substitution which shall deteriorate the quality, commercial value, or medicinal effect, or which shall alter the nature or composition of such drug, medicine, chemical, or pharmaceutical preparation so that it will not correspond to the recognized tests of identity or purity. Any person who shall thus willfully adulterate or alter, or cause to be adulterated or altered, or shall sell or offer for sale, any such drugs, medicine, chemical, or pharmaceutical preparation, or any person who shall substitute, or cause to be substituted, one material for another, with the intention to defraud or deceive the purchaser, shall be guilty of a misdemeanor, and be liable to prosecution under this act. If convicted he shall be liable to all the costs of the action, and for the first offense be liable to a fine of not less than ten dollars nor more than one hundred dollars, and for each subsequent offense a fine of not less than twenty-five dollars nor more than one hundred and fifty dollars. On complaint being entered, the board of pharmacy is hereby empowered to employ an analyst or chemist, whose duty it shall be to examine into the so-called adulteration, substitution, or alteration, and report upon the result of his investigation; and if said report shall be deemed to justify such action, the board shall duly cause the prosecution of the offender, as provided in this act.

SEC. 12. The senior pharmacist of every house dispensing and compounding medicines, registered under this act, shall be exempt and free from all jury duty in the courts of this State.

SEC. 13. All acts and parts of acts in conflict with the provisions of this act are hereby repealed.

Approved June 2, 1885.

NOTE.—Section 10 in this act is the amended section, entitled an "Act to amend section 10," etc. Approved June 18, 1887.

## MINNESOTA.

*Be it enacted by the Legislature of the State of Minnesota:*

"SECTION 1. That except as in this act provided, it shall hereafter be unlawful for any person to retail, compound, or dispense drugs, medicines, or poisons, or to institute or conduct any pharmacy, store, or shop for retailing, compounding, or dispensing drugs, medicines, or poisons, unless such person shall be a registered pharmacist, or shall employ, place, and keep in active charge and control of said pharmacy, store, or shop a registered pharmacist, within the full meaning of this act." (As amended in 1891.)

SEC. 2. To be entitled to registration as a pharmacist within the full meaning of this act the applicant must be a graduate in pharmacy, or a graduate in medicine, within the requirements of this act, or he must be not less than twenty-one (21) years of age, and have had four (4) years' practical experience in drug stores where prescriptions of medical practitioners have been usually compounded, and have sustained a satisfactory examination before the board of pharmacy of the State of Minnesota, or he must be at the time of the passage of this act a registered assistant.

Nothing in this section contained shall impair the validity of any registration heretofore granted by said board. But notwithstanding anything in this section hereinbefore contained, any person who was on the 5th day of March, 1885, entitled to registration as a registered pharmacist, and who is at the time of the passage of this act engaged in the business of a dispensing pharmacist in the State of Minnesota, and who shall within thirty (30) days after the passage of this act file with the secretary of said board an application for registration, accompanied with his affidavit that he was on the 5th day of March aforesaid, as well as at the time of the passage of this act, so engaged, shall be granted a certificate of registration without examination. (As amended in 1891.)

SEC. 3. A graduate in pharmacy or in medicine must, in order to be so registered, have had four (4) years' practical experience in drug stores where prescriptions of medical practitioners have been usually compounded and have a diploma from a college or school of pharmacy or medicine satisfactory to said board of pharmacy, as sufficient guarantee of his attainments and proficiency, or he shall be legally entitled to practice medicine in the State of Minnesota. (As amended in 1891.)

SEC. 4. The said board of pharmacy may, at their discretion, grant registration and a certificate thereof to any pharmacist licensed or registered by the board of pharmacy of any other State, either after or without further examination. It shall be the duty of said board to grant an assistant's certificate to any person not less than eighteen (18) years of age who shall have had two (2) years' practical experience in drug stores where prescriptions of medical practitioners have been usually compounded, and who shall have passed a satisfactory examination before said board of pharmacy of Minnesota; which certificate shall entitle such person to act only as an assistant to a registered pharmacist personally conducting his own business as such, and shall not entitle such assistant to engage in business on his own account, or as manager, to conduct a drug store, or to transact a pharmacy business for another party. (As amended in 1891.)

SEC. 5. Immediately upon the passage of this act the Minnesota State pharmaceutical association shall elect fifteen (15) reputable and practicing pharmacists doing business in the State, from which number the governor shall appoint five (5). The said five (5) pharmacists, duly elected and appointed, shall constitute the board of pharmacy of the State of Minnesota, and shall hold, office as respectively designated in their appointments, for the term of one, two, three, four, and five years, respectively, as hereinafter provided, and until their successors have been duly elected and appointed. The Minnesota State pharmaceutical association shall annually thereafter elect five (5) pharmacists, from which number the governor of the State shall appoint one to fill the vacancy annually occurring in said board. The term of office shall be five years. In case of resignation or removal from the State of any member of said board, or of a vacancy occurring from any cause, the governor shall fill the vacancy by appointing a pharmacist from the names last submitted to serve as a member of the board for the remainder of the term.

SEC. 6. The said board shall, within sixty (60) days after its appointment, meet and organize by the selection of a president and secretary from the number of its own members, who shall be elected for the term of one year, and shall perform the duties prescribed by the board. It shall be the duty of the board to examine all applications for registration submitted in proper form; to grant certificates of registration to such persons as may be entitled to the same under the provisions of this act; to cause the prosecution of all persons violating its provisions; to report annually to the governor and to the Minnesota State pharmaceutical association upon the condition of pharmacy in the State, which said report shall also furnish a record of the proceedings of said board for the year, as well as the names of all pharmacists duly registered under this act. The board shall hold meetings for the examination of applicants for registration and transaction of such other duties as shall pertain to its duties at least once in three months, and the said board shall give thirty (30) days' public notice of the time and place of such meeting. The said board shall also have power to make by-laws for the proper execution of its duties under this act, and shall keep a book of registration, in which shall be entered the names and places of business of all persons registered under this act, which registration book shall also contain such facts as such persons claim to justify their registration. Three members of said board shall constitute a quorum.

SEC. 7. Every person claiming the right of registration under this act, who shall, within three months after the passage of this act, forward to the board of pharmacy satisfactory proof, supported by his affidavit, that he was engaged in the business of dispensing pharmacist on his own account in the State of Minnesota at the time of the passage of this act, as provided in section 2, shall, upon the payment of the fee hereinafter mentioned, be granted a certificate of registration: *Provided*, That in case of failure or neglect to register as herein specified, then such person shall, in order to be registered, comply with the requirements provided for registration as graduates in pharmacy or licentiates in pharmacy within the meaning of this act.

SEC. 8. Any person engaged in the position of assistant in a pharmacy at the time this act takes effect, not less than eighteen years of age, who shall have had at least three (3) years' practical experience in drug stores where the prescriptions of medical practitioners are compounded, and who shall furnish satisfactory evidence to that effect to the State board of pharmacy, shall, upon making application for registration and upon payment to the secretary of said board a fee of one dollar, within ninety (90) days after this act takes effect, be entitled to a certificate as "registered assistant," which certificate shall entitle him to continue in such duties as clerk or assistant; but shall not entitle him to engage in business on his own account. Thereafter he shall pay annually to the said secretary the sum of fifty cents, during the time he shall continue in such duties, in return for which sum he shall receive a renewal of said certificate: *Provided*, Any applicant who has had seven years' experience in compounding and dispensing medicines immediately prior to the passage of this act may receive a certificate of a "registered pharmacist."

SEC. 9 Every person claiming registration as a registered pharmacist under this act shall, before a certificate is granted, pay to the secretary of the board of pharmacy the sum of two (2) dollars; and every applicant for registration upon examination, whether as a pharmacist or as an assistant, shall pay to said secretary the sum of five (5) dollars before such examination shall be attempted: *Provided*, That in case the applicant fails to sustain a satisfactory examination by the said board, the said five (5) dollars shall be refunded to him. Every certificate hereafter issued under this act shall have plainly written, printed, or stamped upon the face thereof the words: "Revocable for the causes specified by law." (As amended in 1891.)

SEC. 10. Every registered pharmacist and every registered assistant who desires to continue the practice of his profession, shall annually during the time he shall continue such practice, on such date as the board of pharmacy may prescribe, pay to said secretary a registration renewal fee, the amount of which shall be fixed by said board, and shall in no case exceed two (2) dollars for a pharmacist, and one (1) dollar for an assistant; in return for which payment he shall receive a renewal of his registration. (As amended in 1891.)

SEC. 11. The secretary of the board of pharmacy shall receive a salary which shall be determined by said board; he shall also receive his traveling and other expenses incurred in the performance of his official duties. The other members of said board shall receive the sum of five dollars for each day actually engaged in such service, and all the legitimate and necessary expenses incurred in attending the meetings of said board. Said expenses shall be paid from the fees, fines, and penalties received by said board under the provisions of this act; and no part of the salary or other expenses of said board shall be paid out of the public treasury. All moneys received by said board in excess of said allowances and other expenses hereinbefore provided for shall be held by the secretary of said board as a special fund for meeting the expenses of said board, said secretary giving such bonds as the said board shall from time to time direct. The said board shall, in its annual report to the governor and to the Minnesota State pharmaceutical association, render an account of all moneys received and disbursed by them pursuant to this act. (As amended in 1891.)

SEC. 12. Any person not being, or not having in his employ a registered pharmacist within the full meaning of this act, who shall, after this act shall take effect, retail, compound, or dispense drugs, medicines, or poisons, or who shall take, use, or exhibit the title of a registered pharmacist, shall for each and every such offense be liable to a penalty of fifty (50) dollars.

Any registered pharmacist or other person who shall permit the compounding or dispensing of prescriptions, or the vending of drugs, medicines, or poisons in his store or place of business, except under the supervision of a registered pharmacist or by a registered assistant, and any pharmacist or registered assistant who, while continuing in business, shall fail or neglect to procure annual registration, and any person who shall willfully make any false representation to procure registration for himself or any other person, or who shall violate any other provision of this act, shall, except as otherwise provided, for each and every such offense be liable to a penalty of fifty (50) dollars.

Except as in this section hereafter provided, drugs, medicines, and poisons shall, for all purposes of this act, be construed to include all substances, animal, vegetable, or mineral, commonly kept in stock in drug stores or apothecary shops, and used in compounding medicines or sold for medicinal purposes.

It is provided, however, that nothing in this act shall in any manner interfere with the regular practice of any physician as such, or prevent him as a physician from supplying to his patients such articles as may seem to him proper, or shall interfere with the making or vending of proprietary medicines, or with the sale by general retail dealers of any of the following articles, that is to say:

| | | |
|---|---|---|
| Alum, | Epsom salts, | Logwood, |
| Blue vitriol, | Glauber salts, | Rolled sulphur, |
| Borax, | Glycerine, | Saltpetre, |
| Carbonate of ammonia, | Gum arabic, | Senna leaves, |
| Carbonate of soda, | Gum camphor, | Sublimed sulphur, |
| Castor oil, | Licorice, | Water of ammonia, |
| Copperas, | | |

or with the sale by such retail dealers of Paris green, kept in stock in sealed packages, and so sold, distinctly labeled "Paris Green, Poison," or shall prevent a shopkeeper whose place of business is more than one mile from a drug store or apothecary shop, from dealing in and selling the commonly used medicines and poisons, if put up for such sale by a registered pharmacist; or interfere with the exclusively wholesale business of any dealers, except as hereinbefore provided. (As amended in 1891.)

SEC. 13. Every proprietor or conductor of a drug store shall be held responsible for the quality of all drugs, chemicals, and medicines sold or dispensed by him, except those sold in the original package of the manufacturer, and except those articles or preparations known as patent or proprietary medicines. Any person who shall knowingly, willfully, or fraudulently falsify or adulterate, or cause to be falsified or adulterated, any drug or medical substance, or any preparation authorized or recognized by the pharmacopœia of the United States, or used or intended to be used in medical practice; or shall mix or caused to be mixed with any such drug or medicinal substance any foreign or inert substance whatsoever, for the purpose of destroying or weakening its medicinal power and effect, or of lessening its cost, and shall willfully, knowingly, or fraudulently sell or cause the same to be sold for medicinal purposes, shall be deemed guilty of a misdemeanor, and upon conviction thereof shall pay a fine not exceeding five hundred dollars, and shall forfeit to the State of Minnesota all articles so adulterated, "and any person so convicted may also, at the discretion of the court before which conviction occurs, be further adjudged and sentenced to forfeit his registration and the certificate thereof." (As amended in 1891.)

SEC. 14. No person shall sell at retail any poisons commonly recognized as such, and especially aconite, arsenic, belladonna, biniodide of mercury, carbolic acid, chloral hydrate, chloroform, conium, corrosive sublimate, creosote, croton oil, cyanide of potassium, digitalis, hydrocyanic acid, laudanum, morphine, nux vomica, oil of bitter almonds, oil tansy, opium, oxalic acid, strychnine, sugar of lead, sulphate of zinc, white precipitate, red precipitate, without affixing to the box, bottle, vessel, or package containing the same, and to the wrapper or cover thereof, a label bearing the name "POISON" distinctly shown, together with the name and place of business of the seller. Nor shall he deliver any of the said poisons to any person without satisfying himself that such poison is to be used for legitimate purposes: *Provided*, That nothing herein contained shall apply to the dispensing of physicians' prescriptions specifying any of the poisons aforesaid.

"Every person omitting to comply with any requirement of this section shall be deemed guilty of a misdemeanor, and shall upon conviction thereof pay a fine not less than (5) dollars for each such omission." (As amended in 1891.)

SEC. 15. All suits for the recovery of the several penalties prescribed in this act shall be prosecuted in the name of the State of Minnesota, in any court having jurisdiction; and it shall be the duty of the county attorney of the county wherein such offense is committed, to prosecute all persons violating the provisions of this act, upon proper complaint being made.

If in any such case the county attorney omit or refuse to act, the board may employ some other attorney for such purpose.

Costs and disbursements shall be adjudged in favor of the State whenever it recovers judgment in such suit. All fines and penalties paid or collected under the provisions of this act shall inure one-half to the board of pharmacy, and the remainder to the school fund of the county in which the conviction was had or the judgment obtained. If any person adjudged liable to any penalty or penalties imposed by this act shall not pay the judgment therefor within sixty (60) days after the rendition thereof, or, in case of appeal, within thirty (30) days after the affirmation of such judgment, his registration and certificate thereof may be by the board of pharmacy summarily revoked and cancelled, and such person shall not be entitled to registration within one year thence next to ensue or without paying such judgment in full. (As amended in 1891.)

SEC. 16. All acts or portions of acts regulating the practice of pharmacy and the sale of poisons, or the adulteration of drugs, within this State, enacted prior to the passage of this act, are hereby repealed: *Provided,* That nothing in this act shall be so construed as to prevent any person who has once been a registered member, and may have forfeited his membership by nonpayment of dues or fees, from renewing his membership within two years, by paying the required dues or fees, without examination.

SEC. 17. All persons registered under this act shall be exempt from jury duty in the State of Minnesota.

SEC. 18. Every person receiving a certificate under this act shall keep the same conspicuously exposed in his place of business. Every registered pharmacist or registered assistant shall, within ten (10) days after changing his place of business or employment, notify the secretary of the board of his new place of business; he shall thereupon be entitled to receive from the secretary a notice in writing that his address has been changed on the book of registration. Without such notice from said secretary, such pharmacist or assistant shall not act as such longer than ten (10) days after his aforesaid notice of change.

Any person violating the provisions of this section shall be deemed guilty of a misdemeanor, and upon conviction thereof shall be punished by a fine of ten (10) dollars and the cost of prosecution.

SEC. 19. Any registration obtained by false representation shall be void, and the board of pharmacy may, after hearing complaint and evidence, revoke any certificate which it may determine to have been so obtained.

SEC. 20. The board may hereafter appoint a secretary who is not a member of the board.

(Sections 18, 19, 20 added in 1891.)

SEC. 21. This act shall take effect and be in force from and after its passage. (No changes in 1891 from 18 to 21.)

*Sec. 15 of amendatory act of 1891.*

SEC. 15. This act shall take effect and be in force from and after November 1st, A. D. 1891.

Approved April 17, A. D. 1891.

NEW PENAL CODE OF THE STATE OF MINNESOTA (AS AMENDED 1891).

SEC. 326. *Apothecary omitting to label drugs, or labeling them wrongly.*—An apothecary or druggist, or a person employed as clerk or salesman by an apothecary or druggist, or otherwise carrying on business as a dealer in drugs or medicines, who, in putting up any drugs or medicines, or making up any prescription, or filling any order for drugs or medicines, willfully, negligently, or ignorantly omits to label the same, or puts any untrue label, stamp, or other designation of contents upon any box, bottle, or other package containing a drug or medicine, or substitutes a different article for any article prescribed or ordered, or puts up a greater or less quantity of any article than that prescribed or ordered, or otherwise deviates from the terms of the prescription or order which he undertakes to follow, in consequence of which human life or health is endangered, is guilty of a misdemeanor.

SEC. 327. *Apothecary selling poison without recording the sale.*—An apothecary or druggist, or a person employed as clerk or salesman by an apothecary or druggist, or any person otherwise carrying on business, who shall sell, or give away, arsenic or its preparations, aconite, belladonna, lead or its preparations, mercury or its preparations, hydrocyanic acid, oxalic acid, copper or its preparations, phosphorus, oil of savin, oil of tansy, morphine, strychnine, laudanum, rough on rats, or cyanide of potassium, without first recording, in a book to be kept for that purpose, the name and residence of the person receiving such poison, together with the kind and quantity of such poison received, except upon the written order or prescription of some practicing physician, is guilty of a misdemeanor. Any person purchasing any of the above-named drugs who shall give the person selling the same a false name for registration, shall, upon conviction thereof, be deemed guilty of a misdemeanor: *Provided,* That this section shall not apply to the sale of Paris green.

SEC. 328. *Refusing to exhibit record.*—A person whose duty it is by the last section to keep a book for recording the sale or gift of poisons who willfully refuses to permit any officer, or person acting under the direction of an officer, to inspect said book upon reasonable demand during ordinary business hours shall, upon conviction thereof, be deemed guilty of a misdemeanor and be punished by a fine not to exceed fifty dollars.

SEC. 329. *Selling poison without label.*—An apothecary or druggist, or a person employed as clerk or salesman by an apothecary or druggist, or any person otherwise carrying on business, who shall sell, or give away, arsenic or its preparations, aconite, belladonna, lead or its preparations, mercury or its preparations, hydrocyanic acid, oxalic acid, copper or its preparations, morphine, phosphorus, oil of savin, oil of tansy, oil of cedar, strychnine, rough on rats, cyanide of potassium, carbolic acid, tincture of nux vomica, fluid extract ergot, fluid extract cotton root, chloroform, chloral hydrate, croton oil, sulphate of zinc, mineral acids, stramonium, conium, opium or its preparations, except paregoric and Dewees's carminative, without attaching to the vial, box, or parcel containing such substance a label with the name and residence of such person, the word "poison," and the name of such article written or printed, or partly written and partly printed, thereon, in plain and legible characters, is guilty of a misdemeanor: *Provided,* That the provisions of this section shall not apply when the sale is made upon the written prescription or order of some practicing physician.

SEC. 330. *Medical prescriptions.*—No person employed in a drug store or apothecary shop shall prepare a medical prescription unless he has served two years' apprenticeship in such store or shop, or is graduate of a medical college or college of pharmacy, except under the direct supervision of some person possessing one of those qualifications; nor shall any proprietor or other person in charge of such a store or shop permit any person not possessing such qualifications to prepare a medical prescription in his store or shop, except under such supervision. A person violating any provisions of this section is guilty of a misdemeanor, punishable by a fine not exceeding one hundred dollars, or by imprisonment in the county jail not exceeding six months; and in case of death ensuing from such violation, the person offending is guilty of a felony, punishable by a fine not less than one thousand dollars nor more than five thousand dollars, or by imprisonment in the State prison not less than two years nor more than four years, or by both such fine and imprisonment.

## MISSISSIPPI.

1. *Duty to obtain license.*—Every person who desires to practice pharmaceutics must obtain license to do so, as hereinafter provided.

2. *Board of examiners created.*—The board of pharmaceutical examiners is hereby created, to consist of five (5) practicing pharmacists, who shall be appointed by the governor and whose term of office shall expire with that of the governor appointing them.

3. *Oath of examiners.*—Each person appointed as a member of the board of pharmaceutical examiners shall qualify by taking the oath prescribed by the constitution of the State officers, and shall file a certificate thereof in the office of the secretary of the State within fifteen (15) days of his appointment.

4. *Organization of examiners.*—After the members of the board of pharmaceutical examiners have qualified, they shall meet at the capitol of the State in pursuance of a call to be made by the governor, and organize by electing a president and secretary of the board, from amongst themselves.

5. *License for examination.*—Every person who desires to practice pharmaceutics must apply in writing to the board of pharmaceutical examiners for a license to do so, and unless exempted by the provision of the chapter, must appear before the board and be examined by it, touching his learning and skill in pharmaceutics, and if he be found to possess sufficent learning and skill therein, and be of good moral character, the board shall immediately issue to him a license to practice pharmaceutics, which shall be signed by each member of the board who attends the examination and approve of the issuing of the license.

6. *Examination: When, where, and how conducted.*—The board of pharmaceutical examiners shall meet at the capitol of the State on the first Tuesday in April of each year, for the purpose of examining applicants for license, and shall remain in session until all applicants for such license have been approved or disapproved. All examinations, except as to character, shall be by and upon written questions and answers, and three (3) members of the board is a quorum for business.

7. *Fee for examination.*—Applicants for license who require to be examined touching their learning and skill in pharmacentics must each pay a fee of five (5) dollars to the board of pharmaceutical examiners, as a condition precedent to the examination, which fee shall be distributed among the members of the board as their compensation in such proportion as the board may allow.

8. *License to existing practitioners of pharmaceutics.*—Each person now engaged in the practice of pharmaceutics in this State is entitled to a license therefor without being examined touching his learning or skill, if he shall apply therefor within six (6) months after this law becomes operative, and shall pay twenty-five (25) cents for each issuance; if such application be made within time prescribed, and the twenty-five cents be paid, the secretary of the board of examiners shall issue to the applicant a license to practice pharmaceutics, which shall be signed in the name of the board by him as secretary.

9. *Temporary license.*—Any member of the board of pharmaceutical examiners may examine applicants orally or in writing, and issue a temporary license to him to practice pharmaceutics, which shall authorize such practice and develop until the next succeeding meeting of the board; but only one temporary license shall be issued to the same applicant.

10. *License must be recorded.*—Every person who receives a license to practice pharmaceutics must file it for record in the office of the clerk of the circuit court of the county in which he resides within thirty days after its issuance, and if he fails to do so he shall thereafter be liable for practicing pharmacy without license, so long as the same shall remain unrecorded. When such license shall be filed the clerk shall record the same in the book in which the license of physicians are recorded, upon the payment to him of the lawful fee, and when recorded the original shall be delivered on demand of the license.

11. *License in lieu of one lost.*—If a license to practice pharmaceutics be issued and become lost or destroyed, the board of examiners may issue another in lieu of it, upon satisfactory proof of the loss or destruction.

12. *Board of examiners must keep a record of their proceedings.*—It is the duty of the board of examiners to cause the secretary to keep a complete record of [its] acts and proceedings, and to preserve all papers, documents, and correspondence received by the board and relating to their duties. Office stationery, blanks, etc., such stationery, books, and forms as may be required by the board of pharmaceutical examiners in the discharge of their duties, shall be furnished it by the board of public contracts.

13. *Members of board may be removed and vacancies filled.*—The governor may remove any or all of the members for pharmaceutical examiners, and appoint any other or others in place of such as may be removed, and may fill by appointment any vacancy that may occur in the board.

LAWS REGULATING THE SALE OF POISONS, THE ADULTERATION OF DRUGS, FOOD, ETC., OF MISSISSIPPI.

*Morphine: Sale of, regulated; scarlet wrapper and label, etc.*—If any druggist, or other person, shall sell, offer for sale, or give away any sulphate, or other preparation, of morphine in any bottle, vial, envelope, or other package, without having the same wrapped in a *scarlet* paper or envelope, and labeled with a scarlet label, lettered in white letters, plainly naming the contents of the bottle, vial, envelope, or package, he shall be guilty of misdemeanor, and on conviction shall be fined not less than ten dollars nor more than fifty dollars.

*The same: Physician's certificate.*—If any druggist, or other person, shall sell or give away any sulphate, or other preparation of morphine, or any opium, or any preparation thereof, without the person buying or receiving the same having, presenting, and leaving with the seller or giver a written certificate, signed by some reputable practicing physician, showing that the same is necessary or proper to the health of the person for whose use the same is desired, naming the person, he shall be guilty of a misdemeanor, and on conviction shall be punished as prescribed in the last section.

*The same: False certificate.*—If any physician shall give a certificate, of the kind mentioned in the last section, which is false, he shall be fined not less than twenty dollars nor more than two hundred dollars, and be imprisoned not less than ten days nor more than three months for each offense.

(2744) *Adulteration of food, drugs, candy, confects, and sweetmeats.*—If any person shall manufacture, sell, or keep, or offer, or exhibit for sale any adulterated food or drug, as defined by law, or if any person shall manufacture, sell, or keep, or offer, or exhibit for sale any candy, confect or sweetmeat, in making which any preparation of lime or other deleterious substance is used, he shall, upon conviction, be fined not exceeding five hundred dollars, or be imprisoned in the county jail not more than six months, or both.

(2841) *Trade marks: Counterfeiting and forging of.*—Every person who shall knowingly and wilfully forge or counterfeit, or cause or procure to be forged or counterfeited, any representation, likeness, similitude, copy, or imitation, of the private stamp, wrappers, or labels usually affixed by any mechanic or manufacturer to, and used by such mechanic or manufacturer on, in, or about the sale of any goods, wares, or merchandise whatsoever, shall be guilty of a misdemeanor, and upon conviction shall be punished by fine not exceeding five hundred dollars, or imprisonment in the county jail not less than three months nor more than one year.

(2842) *The same: Possession of plates, dies, etc., for counterfeiting.*—Every person who shall have in his possession any die, plate, engraving, or printed label, stamp, or wrapper, or any representation, likeness, similitude, copy, or imitation of the private stamp, wrapper or label, usually affixed by any mechanic or manufacturer to, and used by such mechanic or manufacturer on, in, or about the sale of any goods, wares, or merchandise, with intent to use or sell the said die, plate, or engraving, or printed stamp, label, or wrapper, for the purpose of aiding or assisting, in any way whatever, in vending any goods, wares or merchandise, in imitation of or intended to resemble and be sold for the goods, wares, or merchandise of such mechanic or manufacturer, shall be guilty of a misdemeanor, and, upon conviction, be punished by fine not exceeding five hundred dollars, or imprisonment in the county jail not less than three months nor more than one year.

(2843) *The same: Selling articles bearing counterfeit.*—Every person who shall vend any goods, wares, or merchandise having thereon any forged or counterfeit stamp or label, imitating, resembling, or purporting to be the stamp or label of any mechanic or manufacturer, knowing the same to be forged or counterfeited, and resembling or purporting to be imitations of the stamps or labels of such mechanic or manufacturer, without disclosing the fact to the purchaser thereof, shall be guilty of a misdemeanor, and upon conviction shall be punished by imprisonment in the county jail not exceeding three months, or by a fine not less than fifty nor more than five hundred dollars, or both.

*Selling by false weights or measures.*—If any person shall sell anything by any false weight or measure whereby another shall be cheated, or if any person shall sell any light-weight loaf, or package, calling the same a pound or other quantity, or if any person shall sell any under-capacity bottle or other vessel, calling it a pint, quart, or other quantity, he shall be guilty of a misdemeanor, and fined not less than ten dollars, and imprisoned not less than ten days.

*Dealers to have none but sealed measures.*—When the county or city is supplied with the standards of weights and measures, every dealer therein shall have none but sealed weights and measures, and the weights shall be so sealed as that the removal of any part of the filling will destroy or deface the seal; and every dealer having, in such case, any weight or measure which has not been duly sealed shall be guilty of a misdemeanor, and shall, moreover, forfeit ten dollars for every day he may have any unsealed weight or measure.

(2884) *The same: Giving medicine, etc., to pregnant women and thereby killing child.*—Every person who shall administer to any woman pregnant with a quick child any medicine, drug, or substance whatever, or shall use or employ any instrument or other means, with intent thereby to destroy such child, and shall thereby destroy it, shall be guilty of manslaughter, unless the same shall have been necessary to preserve the life of the mother, or shall have been advised by a physician to be necessary for such purpose.

(2892) *The same: Drunken doctors, etc., unintentionally causing death.*—If any physician, or other person, while in a state of intoxication, shall, without a design to effect death, administer, or cause to be administered, any poison, drug, or other medicine, or shall perform any surgical operation on another, which shall cause the death of such other person, he shall be guilty of manslaughter.

(2930) *Poisons: Sales and gifts of, regulated.*—It shall not be lawful for any apothecary, druggist, or other person to sell or give away any articles belonging to the class of medicines usually denominated poisons, except in compliance with the two following sections.

(2631) *The same: Register to be kept, label, etc.*—Every druggist, apothecary, or other person, who shall sell or give away, except upon the written prescription of a physician, any article of medicine belonging to the class usually known as poisons, shall be required to register, in a book kept for that purpose, the name, place of residence, age, sex, and color of the person obtaining such poison, the quantity sold, the purpose for which it was required, the day and date on which it was obtained, and the name and place of abode of the person for whom the article is intended; and he shall carefully mark the word "poison" upon the label or wrapper of each package.

(2932) *The same: Arsenic to be mixed with soot or indigo.*—A druggist, apothecary, or other person shall not sell or give away, except to physicians, any quantity of arsenic less than one pound without first mixing soot or indigo therewith, in the proportion of one ounce of soot or half an ounce of indigo to the pound of arsenic.

(2933) *The same: Penalty for violation of last two sections.*—Any druggist or apothecary, or other person, who shall offend against the provisions of the last section or the one before the last, shall, on conviction, be fined not exceeding five hundred dollars, or imprisoned in the county jail twenty days, or both.

(2934) *The same: Not to be sold to minors.*—A druggist, apothecary, or other person shall not sell or give away any to any minor, and for so doing he shall be punished as for a misdemeanor.

(2935) *The same: Poisoning fish in water.*—Every person who shall poison any fish by mingling in the water any substance calculated and intended to stupefy or destroy fish, shall be guilty of a misdemeanor, and on conviction shall be fined not less than five dollars, or imprisoned in the county jail not less than ten days, or both.

(2936) *The same: Poisoning person with intent to kill, where death does not ensue.*—Every person who shall be convicted of having administered, or of having caused or procured to be administered, any poison to any human being, with intent to kill such human being, and which shall have been actually taken by such human being, whereof death shall not ensue, shall be punished by imprisonment in the penitentiary for a term not less than ten years.

(2937) *The same: Mingling poison with food, drink, or medicine; poisoning spring, well, reservoir of water, etc.*—Every person who shall mingle any poison with any food, drink, or medicine, with intent to kill or injure any human being, or who shall willfully poison any well, spring, or reservoir of water, shall, upon conviction, be punished by imprisonment in the penitentiary not exceeding ten years, or in the county jail not exceeding one year, or by fine not exceeding one thousand dollars, or both.

(2938) *The same: Administering to animals.*—Every person who shall willfully and unlawfully administer any poison to any horse, mare, colt, mule, jack, jennet, cattle, deer, dog, hog, sheep, chicken, goose, turkey, pea-fowl, guinea-fowl, or partridge, or shall maliciously expose any poisonous substance, with intent that the same should be taken or swallowed by any horse, mare, colt, mule, jack, jennet, cattle, dog, hog, sheep, chicken, goose, turkey, pea-fowl, guinea-fowl, or partridge, shall, upon conviction, be punished by imprisonment in the penitentiary not exceeding three years, or in the county jail not exceeding one year, and by a fine not exceeding five hundred dollars.

(2950) *The same: Merchants other than druggists not to open store, etc.*—A merchant, shopkeeper, or other person shall not keep open store, or dispose of any wares or merchandise, goods, or chattels on Sunday, or sell or barter the same; and every person so offending shall, on conviction, be fined not more than twenty dollars for every such offense; but this shall not apply to apothecaries or druggists who may open their stores for the sale of medicines.

(LAWS 1884, p. 82.) *Toy pistols: Sale of, and of cartridges or caps for, prohibited.*—If any person shall sell, or offer or expose for sale, any toy pistol, or cartridges or caps or other contrivance by which such pistols are fired or made to cause an explosion, he shall be guilty of a misdemeanor, and on conviction shall be punished by fine not less than five dollars nor more than twenty-five dollars, or imprisonment in the county jail not less than three days nor more than thirty days, or both.

If the druggist be a dram-shop keeper he can not keep the drug store open if thereby he gives access to the dram-shop. (*See* §. —) Elkin v. State, 63 Miss., 129.

# MISSOURI.

CHAPTER 58, REVISED STATUTES OF MISSOURI, 1889, SECTIONS 4610–4625, INCLUSIVE.

SECTION 4610. *Druggist must be registered.*—It shall be unlawful for any person not a registered pharmacist within the meaning of this chapter, to conduct any pharmacy, drug store, apothecary shop or store, for the purpose of retailing, compounding or dispensing, medicine or poisons for medical use, except as hereinafter provided. (Laws, 1881, p. 130.)

SEC. 4611. *Registered pharmacist to compound, etc.; physicians may register; penalty.*—It shall be unlawful for the proprietor of any store or pharmacy to allow any person, except a registered pharmacist, to compound or dispense the prescriptions of physicians, or to retail or dispense poisons for medical use, except as an aid to and under the supervision of a registered pharmacist: *Provided,* That nothing in this chapter shall be construed to require any physician duly authorized to practice medicine in this State to submit to an examination as a condition precedent to a license as a pharmacist, but that the same shall be issued upon the presentation of his diploma as a physician. Any person violating the provisions of this section shall be deemed guilty of a misdemeanor, and on conviction thereof shall be liable to a fine of not less than twenty-five dollars nor more than one hundred dollars for each and every offense. (Laws, 1881, p. 130, amended.)

SEC. 4612. *Board of pharmacy.*—The governor, with the approval of the senate, shall appoint three persons from among the most competent pharmacists of the State, not connected with any school of pharmacy, all of whom shall have been residents of the State for at least five years, and of at least five years' practical experience in their profession, who shall be known and styled "board of pharmacy for the State of Missouri," one of whom shall hold his office for one year, one for two years, and one for three years, and each until his successor shall be appointed and qualified; and each year thereafter another member shall be appointed for three years, or until his successor be appointed and qualified. If a vacancy occur in said board another shall be appointed, as aforesaid, to fill the unexpired term thereof. Said board shall have power to make by-laws and all necessary regulations, and create auxiliary boards, if necessary, for the proper fulfillment of their duties under this chapter, without expense to the State. (Laws, 1881, p. 130.)

\* \* \* \* \*

12. *Special attention is called to the amendment of section 4613 of the pharmacy law enacted by our last general assembly. Said section now reads (the portion in italics being the amendment):*

\* \* \* \* \* \* \*

SECTION 4613. *Duties of board.*—The board of pharmacy shall register in a suitable book, a duplicate of which shall be kept in the secretary of State's office, the names and places of residence of all persons to whom they issue certificates, and dates thereof; *and no person having received, or who may hereafter receive, a certificate of registration as a pharmacist, shall engage in business as a pharmacist in any county of this State in which he shall locate, or into which he shall afterward remove, until he shall have had such certificate recorded in the office of the clerk of the county court of such county, and it is hereby made the duty of such county clerk to record such certificate in a book to be provided and kept for that purpose; and the county clerk is authorized to charge a fee of 50 cents for the recording of each certificate, to be paid by the person offering such certificate for record.* Every pharmacist now holding a certificate of registration as a pharmacist, and being engaged in business as a pharmacist, shall have such certificate recorded, as is in this section provided, *within thirty days after the taking effect of this act.* The record of each certificate required by this act, or a certified copy thereof, shall be evidence in all courts that the person holding it is a registered pharmacist. Any pharmacist failing to comply with the foregoing provisions shall be deemed guilty of a misdemeanor, and upon conviction thereof shall be fined not less than $25 nor more than $100.

Approved, March 31, 1893.

SEC. 4614. *Examination, how made.*—The said board of pharmacy shall, upon application, and at such time and place and in such manner as they may determine, examine each and every person who shall desire to conduct the business of selling at retail, compounding or dispensing drugs, medicines, or chemicals for medicinal use, or to compound and dispense physicians' prescriptions as pharmacists, and if a majority of said board shall be satisfied that said person is competent and fully qualified to conduct said business of compounding or dispensing drugs, medicines, or chemicals for medicinal use, or to compound and dispense physicians' prescriptions, they shall enter the name of such person as a registered pharmacist in the book provided for in the preceding section; and that all graduates in pharmacy having a diploma from an incorporated college or school of pharmacy, that requires a practical experience in pharmacy of not less than four years before granting diplomas, shall be entitled to have their names registered as pharmacists by said board without examination: *Provided*, That any person not a pharmacist or druggist may own or conduct such store, if he or they keep constantly in his or their employ a competent pharmacist or druggist. (Laws, 1881, p. 130, amended.)

SEC. 4615. *Fees for registration.*—The board of pharmacy shall be entitled to demand and receive, from each person whom they register and furnish a certificate as a registered pharmacist without examination, the sum of one dollar; and for each and every person whom they examine orally, or whose answers to a schedule of questions are returned subscribed on to under oath, the sum of three dollars, which shall be in full for all services; and in case the examination of said person shall prove defective and unsatisfactory, and his name not be registered, he shall be permitted to present himself for reëxamination within any period not exceeding twelve months thereafter, and no charge shall be made for such reëxamination. (Laws, 1881, p. 131.)

SEC. 4616. *Druggist responsible for quality of drugs, etc.*—Every registered pharmacist, apothecary, or owner of any drug store shall be held responsible for the quality of all drugs, chemicals, and medicines he may sell or dispense, with the exception of those sold in original packages of the manufacturer, and also those known as "patent medicines," and should he knowingly, intentionally, and fraudulently adulterate, or cause to be adulterated, such drugs, chemicals, or medical preparations, he shall be deemed guilty of a misdemeanor, and, upon conviction thereof, be liable to a penalty not exceeding one hundred dollars, and, in addition thereto, have his name stricken from the register. (Laws, 1881, p. 131.)

SEC. 4617. *Druggists can sell, what.*—Apothecaries, registered as herein provided, shall have the right to keep and sell, under such restrictions as herein provided, all medicines and poisons authorized by the National American or United States Pharmacopœia as of recognized medical utility, except intoxicating liquors, which shall only be sold by druggists and pharmacists as prescribed by section 4621 of this chapter. (Laws, 1881, p. 131, amended. Laws, 1883, p. 89, amended.)

SEC. 4618. *Selling poisons; conditions, etc.; penalty.*—It shall be unlawful for any person to retail any poisons enumerated in schedules "A" and "B," except as follows: Schedule "A"—Arsenic and its preparations, biniodide of mercury, cyanide of potassium, hydrocyanic acid, strychnia, and all other poisonous vegetable alkaloids and their salts, and the essential oil of bitter almonds. Schedule "B"—Opium and its preparations, except paregoric and other preparations of opium containing less than two grains to the ounce; aconite, belladonna, colchicum, conium, nux vomica, henbane, savin, ergot, cotton root, cantharides, creosote, veratrum, digitalis, and their pharmaceutical preparations, croton oil, chloroform, chloral hydrate, sulphate of zinc, corrosive sublimate, red precipitate, white precipitate, mineral acids, carbolic acid, oxalic acid, without labeling the box, vessel, or paper in which the said poison is contained, and also the outside wrapper or cover, with the name of the article, the word "poison," and the name and place of business of the seller. Nor shall it be lawful for any person to sell or deliver any poisons enumerated in schedules "A" and "B," unless upon due inquiry it be found that the purchaser is aware of its poisonous character, and represents that it is to be used for legitimate purposes. Nor shall it be lawful for any registered pharmacist to sell any poisons included in schedule "A" without, before delivering the same to the purchaser, causing an entry to be made in a book kept for that purpose, stating the date of sale, name and address of purchaser, the name of poison sold, the purpose for which it was represented by the purchaser to be required, and the name of dispenser —such book to be always open for inspection by the proper authorities and to be preserved for at least five years. The provisions of this section shall not apply to the dispensing of poison in not unusual quantities or doses upon the prescription of practitioners of medicine. Nor shall it be lawful for any licensed or registered druggist or pharmacist to retail, sell, or give away any alcholic liquors or compounds as a beverage. Any person violating the provisions of this section shall be deemed guilty of a misdemeanor, and upon conviction thereof shall be fined not less than twenty-five nor more than one hundred dollars. (Laws, 1881, p. 132.)

SEC. 4619. *Making false representations, etc.; penalty.*—Any person who shall procure or attempt to procure registration for himself or for another under this chapter, by making or causing to be made false representations, shall be deemed guilty of a misdemeanor, and shall, upon conviction thereof, be liable to a penalty of not less than twenty-five nor more than one hundred dollars, and the name of the person so fraudulently registered shall be stricken from the register. Any person not a registered pharmacist, as provided for in this chapter, or who shall conduct a store, pharmacy, or place of retailing, compounding, or dispensing drugs, medicines, or chemicals for medical use, or for compounding or dispersing physicians' prescriptions, or who shall take, use, or exhibit the title of "registered pharmacist," shall be deemed guilty of a misdemeanor, and, upon conviction thereof, shall be liable to a penalty of not less than one hundred dollars, except as provided in section 4614. (Laws, 1881, p. 132.)

SEC. 4620. *Chapter shall not apply to, what.*—This chapter shall not apply to physicians putting up their own prescriptions, nor to the sale of proprietary medicines. (Laws, 1881, p. 133.)

SEC. 4621. *May sell or give away in what quantity, when.*—No druggist, proprietor of a drug store, or pharmacist shall, directly or indirectly, sell, give away, or otherwise dispose of alcohol or intoxicating liquors of any kind in any quantity less than four gallons for any purpose, except on a written prescription, dated and signed, first had and obtained from some regularly registered and practicing physician, and then only when such physician shall state in such prescription the name of the person for whom the same is prescribed, and that such intoxicating liquor is prescribed as a necessary remedy: *Provided,* That any druggist or pharmacist may sell or give away, in good faith, any wine for sacramental purposes: *Provided further,* That any druggist may sell alcohol in less quantities than four gallons for art, mechanical, and scientific purposes, but only on a written application signed by a person known to the druggist to be a mechanic, scientist, or artist, in which application shall be stated the purpose for which alcohol is to be used. Any druggist who shall violate any of the provisions of this section, or any person who shall make a false statement in an application for alcohol, shall be deemed guilty of a misdemeanor, and, on conviction shall, for the first offense, be fined not less than one hundred nor more than five hundred dollars, and for a second offense shall, on conviction, in addition to such fine, have his certificate of registration as a pharmacist revoked. (Laws, 1883, p. 89, amended—*a.*)

SEC. 4622. *Prescriptions must be preserved, etc.; penalty for failure.*—Every druggist, proprietor of drug store, or pharmacist shall carefully preserve all prescriptions compounded by him or those in his employ, numbering, dating, and filing them in the order in which they are compounded, and shall produce the same in court or before any grand jury whenever thereto lawfully required, and on failing, neglecting, or refusing so to do, shall be deemed guilty of a misdemeanor, and, on conviction, shall be punished by a fine of not less than fifty nor more than one hundred dollars. (Laws, 1883, p. 89, amended.)

SEC. 4623. *Penalty for making false prescriptions, etc.*—Any physician doing business as a pharmacist or druggist, and owning and operating a drug store or pharmacy, who shall write and permit the filling out at his own drug store or pharmacy of a prescription calling for intoxicating liquor, except the same is for the purpose and under the conditions mentioned in section 4621 of this chapter, shall be guilty of a misdemeanor, and on conviction shall have his certificate of registration as a druggist or pharmacist revoked as part of the judgment of the court, and in addition thereto be fined in a sum not less than one hundred dollars nor more than five hundred dollars. (Laws, 1881, p. 130; amended laws, 1887, p. 182, amended.)

SEC. 4624. *Prescription for intoxicating liquor, when given, etc.; penalty.*—Any physician, or pretended physician, who shall make or issue any prescription to any person for any intoxicating liquors in any quantity, or for any compound of which such liquors shall form a part, to be used otherwise than for medicinal purposes, or who shall issue more than one prescription at the same time to anyone for intoxicating liquors, or for any compound of which such liquors shall become a part, or who shall make or issue any prescription contrary to any existing law, shall be deemed guilty of a misdemeanor, and, upon conviction, be punished by a fine of not less than forty nor more than two hundred dollars. (R. S., 1879, §5476; Laws, 1887, p. 214, amended.)

SEC. 4625. *Intoxicating liquors not to be drunk on premises; penalty.*—Any druggist or dealer in drugs and medicines who shall suffer alcohol or intoxicating liquors to be drunk at or about his place of business, shall be deemed guilty of a misdemeanor, and upon conviction shall be punished by a fine not exceeding two hundred dollars or by imprisonment in the county jail not exceeding six months. (New section.)

## MONTANA.

Governor Rickards, under date of May 31, 1893, informs the Department that there are no pharmaceutical laws in Montana.

## NEBRASKA.

SECTION 1. There shall be established in the State of Nebraska a board, to be styled the Nebraska State board of pharmacy. Said board shall consist of the attorney-general, secretary of State, auditor, treasurer, and commissioner of public lands and buildings, and said board shall appoint five examiners or secretaries, who shall be skillful retail apothecaries of seven years' practical experience, actually engaged in said business in the State of Nebraska, and said secretaries shall assist said board in conducting all examinations hereinafter provided for, and in the performance of any of its duties. Each of said secretaries shall receive a compensation of five dollars ($5.00) per day for each day's service actually and necessarily performed and such necessary expenses as shall be audited and found just and reasonable by said board for attending the meeting thereof, said secretaries or examiners to be selected from ten practical pharmacists recommended by the Nebraska State pharmaceutical association: *Provided,* That all such services and expenses, and all the necessary expenses of said board shall be paid out of the money received by said board for fees. All moneys received in excess of said per diem allowance, and all other expenses above provided for, shall be paid into the State treasury at the end of each year, and so much thereof as shall be necessary to meet the current expenses of said board shall be subject to the order thereof if, in any year, the receipts of said board shall not be equal to its expenses. The board shall make an annual report, and render account to the State auditor and to the Nebraska State pharmaceutical association of all moneys received and disbursed by it pursuant to this act. And the State of Nebraska shall in no case be liable for any such compensation or expenses: *And provided further*, That said board shall have power to discharge any of said secretaries at any time and to fill any vacancy in the position of secretary whenever from any cause such vacancy exists.

SEC. 2. The said board of examiners shall, within thirty days after its appointment, meet and organize by the election of a president, a secretary, and treasurer from its own members, who shall be elected for the term of one year and serve until their successors are elected and qualified and to perform all the duties prescribed by the board. It shall be the duty of the board to examine all applications for registration submitted in proper form, by such persons as may be entitled to the same under the provisions of this act; to investigate complaints when properly presented, and to cause the prosecution of all persons violating its provisions; to report annually to the governor and to the Nebraska State pharmaceutical association upon the condition of pharmacy in the State, which said report shall also furnish a record of the proceedings of the said board for the year, and also the name of all the pharmacists registered under this act. The board shall hold meetings for the examination of applicants for registration and the transaction of such other business as shall pertain to its duties at least four times a year, said meetings to be held the second Wednesday in February, May, August, and November in each year; and shall make by-laws for the proper fulfillment of its duties; and shall keep a book of registration, in which shall be entered the names and places of business of all persons registered under this act, which book shall also specify such facts as said persons shall claim to justify their registration. The record of said board, or a copy of any part thereof, certified by the secretary to be a true copy, attested by the seal of the board, shall be accepted as competent evidence in all courts of the State. Three members of said board shall constitute a quorum. The president of said board of examiners shall retire from the said board each year and cease to be a member of said board of examiners at the expiration of his term of office. The Nebraska State pharmaceutical association shall annually select three pharmacists from which number the Nebraska State board of pharmacy shall select one to fill vacancy occurring each year.

SEC. 3. Every person who shall, within three months after the passage of this act takes effect, forward to the board of pharmacy satisfactory proof, supported by his affidavit, that he was engaged in the business of a dispensing pharmacist on his own account in this State at the time this act takes effect, in the preparation of physicians' prescriptions, or that at such time he had been employed or engaged three years or more as a pharmacist in the compounding of physicians' prescriptions, and was at said time so employed in this State, shall, upon payment to the board of a fee of two dollars ($2.00), be granted the certificate of registered pharmacist: *Provided*, That in case of failure or neglect to register as herein provided, such person or persons shall, in order to be registered, comply with the requirements provided for registration as a licentiate in pharmacy hereinafter described.

SEC. 4. No other than a licentiate in pharmacy shall be entitled to registration as a pharmacist except as provided in section 3. Licentiates in pharmacy in the meaning of this act shall be such persons, not less than eighteen years of age, who shall have had not less than three years' practical experience in pharmacy, and who shall have passed a satisfactory examination touching their competency before the board of examiners. Every such person shall, before examination is granted, furnish satisfactory evidence that they are of temperate habits, and pay to the board a fee of five dollars: *Provided*, That in case of the failure of any applicant to pass a satisfactory examination, the money shall be held to his credit for a second examination at any time within a year. The said board may grant certificates of registration without further examination to the licentiates of such other boards of pharmacy and graduates of such colleges of pharmacy as it may deem proper upon the payment of five dollars ($5.00), which shall be good only until the first regular meeting of the board thereafter. Licentiates in pharmacy shall at the time of passing their examination be registered by the secretary of State board of examiners as registered pharmacists.

SEC. 5. Assistants who have held a certificate of registration in this State for two consecutive years may, upon application to the board of examiners, be granted a certificate as a registered pharmacist by paying a fee of three dollars: *Provided*, That the applicant has been continually in the practice of pharmacy for two years next preceding his registration as an assistant.

SEC. 6. Every registered pharmacist who desires to continue the practice of his profession shall annually after the expiration of the first year of his registration during the time he shall continue in such practice, on or before the 24th day of March of each year, pay to the said board a registration fee of two dollars ($2.00), for which he shall receive a renewal of said registration. Every person receiving a certificate under this act shall keep the same conspicuously exposed in his place of business. Every registered pharmacist shall, after changing his place of business or employment, as designated by his certificate, notify the secretary of the board of his new place of business. If any pharmacist shall fail or neglect to procure his annual registration or comply with the other provisions of this section, his right to act as such pharmacist shall cease at the expiration of ten days from the time of notice of such failure to comply with the provisions of this section shall have been mailed to him by the secretary of said board, and such pharmacist shall be barred from the practice of pharmacy until he shall have made application and passed the examination provided for in section 4 of this act.

SEC. 7. Any registration obtained through false representations shall be void, and the board of pharmacy may hear complaints and evidence and may revoke such certificates as it may deem improperly held.

SEC. 8. Any proprietor of a pharmacy who, not being a registered pharmacist, or any such proprietor who shall, by himself or any person, permit the compounding or dispensing of prescriptions or vending of drugs, medicines, or poisons in his store or place of business, except by or in the presence of or in and under the supervision of a registered pharmacist; who shall retail, compound, or dispense drugs, poisons, or medicines of any kind, or any person violating any provisions of this act to which no other penalty is herein attached, shall be deemed guilty of a misdemeanor, and for every such offense, and upon conviction thereof, shall be punished by a fine of not less than ten dollars nor more than $100,000, [$100?] or shall be imprisoned not less than ten days nor more than ninety days: *Provided*, That nothing in this act shall be construed so as to prohibit a registered pharmacist from taking an apprentice to learn the business of pharmacy.

SEC. 9. Nothing in this act shall prevent any wholesale or retail dealers in any business from selling any patent or proprietary medicines, nor any resident registered physician from dispensing his own medicines on his own prescriptions.

SEC. 10. No person shall add to or remove from any drug, medicine, chemical, or pharmaceutical preparation any ingredient or material for the purpose of adulteration or substitution which shall deteriorate the quality, value, or medical effect, or which shall alter the nature or composition of such drug, medicine, chemical, or pharmaceutical preparation, so that it will not correspond to the recognized tests of identity or purity. Any person who shall thus willfully adulterate or alter, or cause to be adulterated or altered, or shall offer for sale any such drug, medicine, chemical, or pharmaceutical preparation, or any person who shall substitute or cause to be substituted one material for another, with the intention to defraud or deceive the purchaser, shall be guilty of a misdemeanor and be liable to prosecution under this act. If convicted he shall be liable to all the costs of the action, and for the first offense be liable to a fine of not less than ten dollars ($10.00) or more than one hundred dollars ($100.00), and for each subsequent offense a fine of not less than twenty-five dollars ($25.00) or more than one hundred dollars ($100.00). On complaint being entered, the board of pharmacy is hereby empowered to employ an analyst or chemist whose duty it shall be to examine into the so-called adulteration, substitution, or alteration and report upon the result of his investigation, and if the said report shall be deemed to justify such action, the board shall duly cause the prosecution of the offender as provided in this act.

SEC. 11. All suits for the recovery of the penalties prescribed in this act shall be prosecuted in the name of the State of Nebraska in any court having jurisdiction, and it shall be the duty of the prosecuting attorney of the county where such offense has been committed to prosecute all persons violating the provisions of this act upon proper complaint being made to them.

SEC. 12. The pharmacist of every house dispensing and compounding medicines registered under this act shall be exempt and free from jury duty in the courts of this State.

SEC. 13. That said sections 2, 4, 5, 6, and 8 of article 3, chapter 52, laws of 1887, as now existing, be, and the same are hereby, repealed.

SEC. 14. Whereas, there being an emergency, this act shall take effect and be in full force from and after its passage.

DECISIONS OF THE ATTORNEY-GENERAL ON THE NEBRASKA PHARMACY LAW.

ATTORNEY-GENERAL'S OFFICE,
Lincoln, May 22, 1889.

Mr. JAMES REED,
    Nebraska City, Nebr.:

DEAR SIR: In answer to your letter of 20th, asking if a grocer violates the pharmacy law by selling sulphur and copperas, I will say that the section of the law provides if any person not being a registered pharmacist shall retail, compound, or dispense drugs, poisons, or medicines he violates the law. If the articles above mentioned are drugs, then a grocer can not legally sell them without being a registered pharmacist. I do not fully know the use that such articles can be put to, and therefore can not see where the harm will be in allowing a grocer to sell them. If they are drugs then the sale is prohibited. I think that it would be a good thing to test the question. As a drug is defined, any commodity used for medicine, dyeing, tanning, and various other purposes, and if the articles sold are used for these purposes, then I am inclined to think there is a violation of the law.

Yours, etc.,

WM. LEESE,
Attorney-General.

Mr. HENRY D. BOYDEN,
    Grand Island, Nebr.:

DEAR SIR: In answer to yours of the 19th inst. I will say that I do not think any person is entitled to a druggist's permit to sell liquors or any other drugs or medicines unless he is registered. A druggist's permit is only granted to druggists, and it would be an evasion of the liquor law to allow a drug store to keep a barroom.

If a druggist is not registered he can not legally sell drugs, and if he has drugs that he can not sell and sells only liquor he is a saloon-keeper, and the keeping of drugs is a sham. The liquors are to be sold only for certain purposes named, and then must be by a druggist.

Yours, etc.,

WM. LEESE,
Attorney-General.

## NEVADA.

Has no pharmacy law.

## NEW HAMPSHIRE.

CHAPTER 135.—SALE OF DRUGS AND MEDICINES.

SECTION 1. No person shall conduct or keep a shop of any kind in this State for the purpose of retailing drugs, medicines, or such chemicals as are used in compounding medicines, or engage in the business of compounding and putting up prescriptions of physicians and selling medicines, either as a proprietor, agent, or assistant, without having first obtained a certificate from the commissioners appointed under the provisions of this chapter; but it shall be lawful for any person to sell proprietary medicines, or to be an owner in the stock in trade in any druggist or apothecary's shop, if he takes no part in conducting or keeping the shop.

SEC. 2. There shall be a commission styled the commission of pharmacy and practical chemistry, which shall be composed of three commissioners, appointed by the governor with the advice of the council, each of whom shall hold his office for three years, and until his successor is appointed and qualified. In case a vacancy shall occur at any time from any cause the governor, with advice of the council, shall fill the vacancy for the unexpired part of the term. The commission as now constituted is continued, subject to the provisions of this chapter.

SEC. 3. The commission shall hold meetings for the examination of applicants for registration, granting of certificates, and the transaction of other necessary business at least quarterly, and at such time and place as they may see fit.

SEC. 4. They shall examine any person desiring to engage in the business of apothecary and druggist, and, if found skilled and learned in pharmacy, shall give to him a certificate stating that he is a skilled pharmacist and authorized to engage in the business of apothecary and druggist.

SEC. 5. They shall examine all applicants over eighteen years of age who have served two years under a registered pharmacist, and grant to such as pass satisfactory minor examinations a certificate as "registered assistant." Such certificate shall not entitle the holder to act as manager of a drug store or pharmacy.

SEC. 6. The commissioners shall procure and keep a suitable book at the office of the secretary of State, wherein they shall register the names and places of residence of all persons to whom they shall issue certificates, and the dates thereof, which shall be open to the examination of all persons at all reasonable times.

SEC. 7. The commission shall file with the secretary of State, on or before the first day of December in each year, a report to the governor and council upon the condition of pharmacy in the State and containing a record of their acts and proceedings.

SEC. 8. Each applicant for a pharmacist's certificate shall pay to the commission a fee of five dollars, and each applicant for a registered assistant's certificate a fee of two dollars, for the use of the board. Each commissioner shall also receive five dollars per day for actual service for not exceeding fifteen days annually, and all necessary expenses incurred in the discharge of his duty, to be paid from the State treasury.

SEC. 9. All pharmacists lawfully registered are authorized to keep spirituous liquors for compounding their medicines.

SEC. 10. If any person shall engage in the business of retailing and vending, directly or indirectly, drugs, medicines, and chemicals, and in dispensing medicine and compounding physicians' prescriptions, without being registered as provided by this chapter or the law heretofore in force, he shall be punished by a fine not exceeding fifty dollars for each week he shall continue the business without being so registered.

SEC. 11. The provisions of this chapter shall not be so construed as to apply to physicians compounding and putting up their own prescriptions.

Passed to take effect Aug. 16, 1889.

## NEW JERSEY.

### CHAPTER CXXIII.

AN ACT to regulate the practice of pharmacy in the State of New Jersey.

SEC. 1. *Be it enacted by the Senate and General Assembly of the State of New Jersey,* That from and after the passage of this act it shall not be lawful for any person not a registered pharmacist within the meaning of this act to conduct any store or pharmacy for retailing, dispensing, or compounding drugs, medicines, or poisons, or for any one not a registered pharmacist to prepare and dispense physicians' prescriptions, or to retail or dispense medicines or poisons, except under the immediate supervision of a registered pharmacist.

SEC. 2. *And be it enacted,* That on or before the first day of June next the New Jersey pharmaceutical association shall submit to the governor the names of fifteen pharmacists doing business within this State, from which number the governor shall appoint five persons, who shall constitute the board of pharmacy of the State of New Jersey, and who shall hold office for the terms of one, two, three, four, and five years, as designated in their respective appointments, and until their successors shall have been appointed and qualified. The New Jersey pharmaceutical association shall annually thereafter nominate to the governor five pharmacists, of whom the governor shall appoint one to fill the vacancy annually occurring in the said board, who shall hold office for five years and until his successor shall have been appointed and qualified. Any vacancy occurring in said board shall be filled by the governor for the unexpired term from among the persons last nominated to him. Each person so appointed shall, within thirty days after appointment, take and subscribe an oath, before any officer authorized to administer oaths in the State, that he will faithfully and impartially discharge the duties prescribed by this act.

SEC. 3. *And be it enacted,* That the board of pharmacy shall organize by electing a president, a secretary, and a treasurer, and shall have power to make by-laws and rules for the proper fulfillment of its duties under this act; it shall meet at least once in three months alternately in the cities of Paterson, Newark, Trenton, and Camden, and shall give thirty days' notice of the time and place of such meetings; it shall examine into all applications for registration, and grant certificates of registration to pharmacists having diplomas from colleges of pharmacy, or regularly chartered medical colleges, granted on four years' practical experience, and to such other persons as it shall judge, on examination, to be properly qualified to practice pharmacy; it shall keep a book of registration, in which shall be entered the names and places of business of all persons registered under this act, and shall also keep a book of record of all its official transactions, which book shall be legal evidence of such transactions in any court of law; it shall have power to examine into all cases of alleged abuses, fraud, and incompetence, cause the prosecution of all persons not complying with the provisions of this act, and suspend and revoke the registration of any person legally convicted of violating the same; it shall report annually to the governor and to the president of the New Jersey pharmaceutical association upon the condition of pharmacy in the State, which report shall embrace a detailed statement of the receipts and expenditures of the board; the members of such board shall receive the sum of five dollars for each day actually engaged in this service, to be paid from the fees and penalties collected under the provisions of this act, and all moneys thus collected by said board in excess of said per diem allowance and of the necessary expense of said board, shall be paid to the treasurer of the New Jersey pharmaceutical association at its annual meeting; three members of the board shall constitute a quorum.

SEC. 4. *And be it enacted,* That every person applying for registration under this act shall furnish satisfactory evidence that he has had at least four years' experience in the practice of pharmacy, and pay to the treasurer of the board of pharmacy a fee of five dollars, and, upon passing an examination satisfactory to said board, he shall receive from said board a certificate of registration; in case of failure to pass a satisfactory examination, the applicant shall be granted a second examination (without the payment of another fee) at any time within six months from his first examination; the registration fee to pharmacists having the diplomas mentioned in section three shall be two dollars; every pharmacist owning or conducting a pharmacy or store shall conspicuously display his certificate of registration in said pharmacy or store, and any failure to do so shall be prima facie evidence that such person is not a registered pharmacist.

SEC. 5. *And be it enacted,* That any person who shall procure or attempt to procure registration for himself or any other person under this act, by making or causing to be made any false representations, or fraudulently represent himself to be registered, or shall adulterate or sell any adulterated drug, medicine, or chemical, or who shall otherwise violate the provisions of this act (except section six), shall be deemed guilty of a misdemeanor and, upon conviction thereof, be liable to a penalty of not less than fifty or more than one hundred dollars, and for every subsequent offense or offenses a like fine, or imprisonment not to exceed six months, or both, at the discretion of the court.

SEC. 6. *And be it enacted,* That it shall not be lawful for any person to retail or dispense any of the poisons enumerated in schedule A appended to this section, or any other substance commonly recognized as a deadly poison, without distinctly labeling with a red label the bottle, box, vessel, or wrapper in which such poison is contained with the name of the article, the word "poison," and the name and place of business of the dispenser, nor without being satisfied that the purchaser is aware of its poisonous nature and intends to use it for a legitimate purpose; any person failing to comply with the requirements of this section shall be deemed guilty of a misdemeanor, and for every such omission shall be liable to a fine of not less than ten dollars; and any person who shall give a fictitious name, or who shall make any false representation to the seller when buying any of the poisons thus enumerated, shall be deemed guilty of misdemeanor and be liable to a fine of not less than ten dollars; the penal provisions of this act shall not apply to the sale of such poisons as are used in the arts, agriculture, or in manufacturing, to persons known to be engaged in such pursuits, nor to the dispensing of poisons upon the prescription of a practicing physician.

### SCHEDULE A.

Arsenic and its compounds or chemical derivatives; corrosive sublimate and other poisonous derivatives of mercury; phosphorus and its poisonous derivatives; prussic acid and its poisonous derivatives; tartrate of antimony; essential oil of bitter almonds; oils of tansy, savin, or croton; chloroform, chloral hydrate, aconite, belladonna, conium, cantharides, digitalis, hyoscyamus, nux vomica, Indian hemp, veratrum viride, yellow jessamine, opium, their alkaloids or other preparations (except paregoric and other preparations of opium having less than two grains to the ounce); ergot, savin, cotton root, and their preparations.

SEC. 7. *And be it enacted,* That nothing in this act shall be construed to apply to or in any manner interfere with the strictly professional pursuits of any physician, nor with the making or vending of patent or proprietary medicines, nor with the sale of simple domestic remedies by retail dealers in rural districts one-half mile or more remote from a regular pharmacist, nor with the ownership of any pharmacy or store in part or whole by any person not a registered pharmacist: *Provided,* Such pharmacy or store be at all times in charged of a registered pharmacist; and any person holding a certificate of registration granted under any former act shall be considered a registered pharmacist within the meaning of this act.

SEC. 8. *And be it enacted,* That each and every fine imposed under this act shall be paid to the treasurer of the board of pharmacy.

SEC. 9. *And be it enacted,* That this act shall be a public act and shall take effect immediately: *Provided,* That the organization of the board, as prescribed in section three hereof, may be had and effected at any time within thirty days from the date of the appointment of its members by the governor.

SEC. 10. *And be it enacted,* That all acts and parts of acts conflicting with this act are hereby repealed.

Approved April 5, 1886.

# NEW MEXICO.

### AN ACT regulating the sale of drugs, medicines, and poisons.

*Be it enacted by the Legislative Assembly of the Territory of New Mexico:*

SECTION 1. That from and after the passage of this act it shall be unlawful for any person, not a registered pharmacist within the meaning of this act, to conduct any drug store, pharmacy, apothecary shop or store for the purpose of retailing, compounding, or dispensing medicines in the Territory of New Mexico, except as hereinafter provided.

SEC. 2. That it shall be unlawful for the proprietor of any such store or pharmacy to allow any person, except a registered pharmacist, to compound or dispense the prescriptions of physicians, except as an aid to, and under the supervision of, a registered pharmacist.

Any person violating the provisions of this section shall be deemed guilty of a misdemeanor, and on conviction shall be liable to a fine of not less than five nor more than one hundred dollars.

SEC. 3. The governor shall appoint five persons, all of whom shall have been residents of the Territory for three (3) or more years and of at least eight (8) years' practical experience as druggists or pharmacists, who shall be known and styled "the board of pharmacy" for the Territory of New Mexico, one of whom shall hold the office for five (5) years; one for four (4) years; one for three (3) years; one for two (2) years; one for one (1) year in the first instance; and thereafter the governor shall annually appoint one (1) person, to serve as a member of the board for five (5) years. The persons so appointed shall constitute the board of pharmacy and shall hold the office for the term for which they were appointed, or until their successors are duly appointed and qualified. They, the said board, and each of them, shall, within ten (10) days after their appointment, or being apprised of the same, take and subscribe the usual official oath, before a properly qualified officer of the county in which they reside. The said board shall organize within thirty (30) days from and after their appointment, and annually thereafter, by the election of a president and secretary. A majority of the board shall constitute a quorum for the transaction of business. Said board shall have the power to make by-laws and all necessary regulations for the proper fulfillment of their duties under this act, without expense to the Territory. Any vacancy occurring in said board shall be filled by an appointment by the governor for the unexpired term.

SEC. 4. The board of pharmacy shall register, in a suitable book, a duplicate of which shall be kept in the office of the secretary of the Territory, the names and places of residence of all persons to whom they issue certificates and the dates thereof.

It shall be the duty of said board of pharmacy to register, without examination, as registered pharmacists, all druggists and pharmacists who are engaged in business in the Territory of New Mexico at the passage of this act, as owners, principals, or clerks of stores for retailing, compounding, or dispensing drugs, medicines, or chemicals for medicinal use, or for compounding and dispensing physicians' prescriptions: *Provided*, No druggist's clerk shall be so registered unless he be eighteen (18) years of age and has been engaged in some store or pharmacy where physicians' prescriptions were compounded and dispensed for the space of three (3) years next preceding the passage of this act.

In case of the failure or neglect of any person to apply for registration within sixty (60) days after the organization of the said board of pharmacy, he shall have forfeited the privilege of registering without examination, and he shall only be registered after examination, as set forth in section 5 of this act.

SEC. 5. That the said board of pharmacy shall, upon application, and at such time and place and in such manner as they may determine, examine each and every person who shall desire to conduct the business of selling at retail, compounding, or dispensing drugs, medicines, or chemicals for medical use, or compounding or dispensing physicians' prescriptions as pharmacists in the Territory of New Mexico; and if a majority of said board shall be satisfied that said person is competent and fully qualified to conduct said business of compounding or dispensing drugs, medicines, or chemicals for medical use, or to compound and dispense physicians' prescriptions, they shall enter the name of such person as a registered pharmacist, in the book provided for in section 4 of this act: *Provided*, That all graduates in pharmacy having a diploma from an incorporated college or school of pharmacy that requires a practical experience in pharmacy of not less than three (3) years before granting a diploma may, in the discretion of the board, be entitled to have their names registered as registered pharmacists by said board without examination.

The board of pharmacy shall issue an appropriate certificate to each person registered, which certificate must be conspicuously displayed in every store or place described in this section. Said certificate must be renewed twelve (12) months after each date of issue.

SEC. 6. The board of pharmacy shall be entitled to demand and receive each person whom they register and furnish a certificate as a registered pharmacist, without examination, the sum of two dollars, and for each and every person whom they examine the sum of five dollars, which shall be in full for all services. In case the examination of said person shall prove defective and unsatisfactory to the board, and he be declined registration, he shall be permitted to present himself for reëxamination within twelve (12) months thereafter, and no charge shall be made for such examination.

SEC. 7. The board of pharmacy shall hold quarterly sessions per annum at such times and places as the board may determine; other sessions of the board may also be held whenever and wherever a quorum of the board is present.

In the interim of the sessions of the board, and upon satisfactory evidence of a fitness of an applicant, any one (1) member of the board may, in his discretion, issue a temporary certificate, which shall authorize and empower the holder to conduct a drug store or pharmacy, as set forth in section 5 of this act. Such temporary certificate must be signed by one (1) member, and shall expire and terminate at the date of the next succeeding quarterly session of the board after the granting thereof. No fee shall be demanded for this temporary certificate.

SEC. 8. Every owner of a drug store in the Territory of New Mexico shall be held responsible for the quality of all drugs, chemicals, and medicines he may sell or dispense, with the exceptions of those sold in the original packages of the manufacturer or wholesale dealer, and also those known as proprietary medicines. And should he knowingly, intentionally, and fraudulently adulterate, or cause to be adulterated, such drugs, chemicals, or medical preparations, he shall be deemed guilty of a misdemeanor, and, upon conviction thereof his license as a registered pharmacist shall be thereby revoked, and in addition thereto be liable to a penalty not exceeding five hundred (500) dollars.

SEC. 9. Any person who shall procure or attempt to procure registration for himself or for another under this act, by making or causing to be made false representations, shall be deemed guilty of a misdemeanor, and shall, upon conviction thereof, be liable to a penalty of not less than five and not exceeding one hundred dollars, and his name, together with the name of the person so falsely registered, shall be stricken from the register.

SEC. 10. Any person not a registered pharmacist, as provided in this act, who shall conduct a store or pharmacy, or place for retailing, compounding, or dispensing drugs, medicines, or chemicals, for medical use, or for compounding or dispensing physicians' prescriptions in the Territory of New Mexico, or who shall take, use, or exhibit the title of registered pharmacist, shall be deemed guilty of a misdemeanor, and, upon a conviction thereof, be liable to a penalty of not less than five nor more than one hundred dollars: *Provided*, That any person or persons not a registered pharmacist may own and conduct such store, if he or they keep constantly in their employ a registered pharmacist: *Provided, further*, This act shall not apply to physicians putting up their own prescriptions, nor to the sale of patent or proprietary medicines, nor to the sale of those articles commonly known as "grocers' drugs," except these articles that are denominated "poisons" under the law known as the "New Mexico poison law."

SEC. 11. If any registered pharmacist shall go out of the drug business, and remain out for a period of twelve (12) months, his certificate as registered pharmacist shall thereupon expire.

SEC. 12. All suits for the recovery of the several penalties prescribed in this act shall be prosecuted in the name of "The Territory of New Mexico," in any court having jurisdiction; and it shall be the duty of the prosecuting attorney of the county where such offense is committed to prosecute all persons violating the provisions of this act, upon proper complaint being made. All penalties collected under the provision of this act shall inure to the expense fund of the board which may occur.

SEC. 13. All persons registered under this act shall be exempt and free from all jury duty in the Territory of New Mexico, upon such person making affidavit that there is no other drug store in the town except theirs, and that they have no proper assistant, and can procure no such assistant to attend to their business during their absence.

SEC. 14. It shall be the duty of the said board to grant to persons or merchants in towns or camps having no drug store, minor certificates without charge as they may deem proper, to vend such medicines, compounds, or chemicals as are required by the general public: *Provided*, That this law is not to be so construed as to prevent ranchmen or miners, not within reach of a store or place where drugs are sold, from dispensing medicines to their families or employes: *Provided, further*, That it shall be the duty of the secretary of said board to render an accurate annual statement to the governor of the Territory of all moneys received and expended by said board during each year, and he shall also report upon the general condition of pharmacy throughout the Territory.

SEC. 15. All acts and parts of acts in conflict with this act be, and the same are hereby, repealed. This act shall be in force and take effect from and after its passage.

Approved, February 15, 1889.

## NEW YORK.

CHAPTER 410, OF THE LAWS OF 1882, NEW YORK CITY CONSOLIDATION ACT OF EIGHTEEN HUNDRED AND EIGHTY-TWO. PASSED JULY 1, 1882.

### CHAPTER XXV.

*Title 6.—Pharmacists and druggists.\**

SECTION 2015 (as amended by L. 1889, ch. 448). It shall be unlawful for any person, unless a registered pharmacist, known as a graduate in pharmacy, or as a licentiate in pharmacy within the meaning of this title, to open or conduct any pharmacy or store for retailing, dispensing, or compounding medicines or poisons in the city or county of New York except as hereinafter provided: *Provided*, That the widow or legal representatives of a deceased person, who was a registered pharmacist, known as a graduate in pharmacy or as a licentiate in pharmacy within the meaning of this title, may continue the business of such deceased pharmacist, provided that the actual retailing, dispensing, or compounding of medicines or poisons be only by a graduate in pharmacy or a licentiate in pharmacy, within the meaning of this title.

SEC. 2016. Any person, in order to be registered, shall be either a graduate in pharmacy or a licentiate in pharmacy, or a graduate having a diploma from some legally constituted medical college or society.

---

\* NOTE.—The succeeding ten sections are a reënactment, with slight verbal changes, of sections 1–10 of chapter 817 of the laws of 1872.

SEC. 2017. Graduates of pharmacy, within the meaning of this title, shall be those persons who have had at least four years' experience in stores where prescriptions of medical practitioners have been compounded, and who have obtained a diploma from any college of pharmacy within the United States, or from some authorized foreign institution or examining board; and licentiates in pharmacy shall be those persons who have had at least four years' experience in stores where prescriptions of medical practitioners are compounded, and who shall have passed an examination either before the board for the examination of and licensing druggists and prescription clerks in the city of New York, established by an act passed March twenty-eight, one thousand eight hundred and seventy-one, or before the board of pharmacy created by chapter eight hundred and seventeen of the laws of eighteen hundred and seventy-two, and continued by this title, or such foreign pharmacists as shall present satisfactory credentials or certificates of their competency and qualifications to the said board of pharmacy. Junior assistants or apprentices in pharmacy shall not be permitted to prepare physicians' prescriptions until they have become graduates or licentiates in pharmacy.

SEC. 2018. The members of the College of Pharmacy of the City of New York shall, on the first Monday of April, one thousand eight hundred and eighty-four, and on the same day every third year thereafter, at a special meeting held for that purpose, elect five competent pharmacists, three of whom shall be graduates of some legally constituted medical college, and the remaining two graduates of some legally constituted college of pharmacy of the city of New York, and who shall form and be known as the board of pharmacy. The members of this board shall, within thirty days after their election as aforesaid, individually take and subscribe, before the clerk of the county of New York, an oath faithfully and impartially to discharge the duties prescribed for them by this title. They shall hold office for the term of three years and until their successors are duly elected and qualified; and in case of any vacancy, the trustees of the College of Pharmacy shall fill the same from two or more nominees elected at a special meeting of the college of pharmacy. The said board shall organize for the transaction of business by the election, by them, from their number, for the whole term, of a president and secretary. The board shall meet at least once every three months, and three members shall constitute a quorum. The duties of the said board shall be to transact all business pertaining to the legal regulation of the practice of pharmacy in the city of New York, and to examine and register pharmacists. Any pharmacist applying for examination shall pay to the secretary a fee of five dollars, and should he pass such examination satisfactorily he shall be furnished with a certificate as to his competency and qualifiation, signed by the said board of pharmacy.

SEC. 2019. It shall be the duty of the secretary to keep a book of registration at some convenient place, of which due notice shall be given through the public press, in which book shall be entered, under the supervision of the said board, the names and places of business of all persons coming under the provisions of this title. It shall be the duty of all such persons to appear before the said board of registration, and the fee for the registration of pharmacists shall not exceed two dollars, and for assistants shall not exceed one dollar. The secretary shall give receipts for all moneys received by him, and pay over the same to the treasurer of the College of Pharmacy aforesaid, taking his receipt therefor, which moneys shall be used for the purpose of defraying the expenses of the board of pharmacy, and any surplus shall be for the benefit of the College of Pharmacy. The salary of the secretary shall be fixed by the board, and shall be paid out of the registration fees.

SEC. 2020. Every registered pharmacist shall be held responsible for the quality of all drugs, chemicals, and medicines he may sell or dispense, with the exception of those sold in the original packages of the manufacturer, and also those known as "patent medicines," and should he knowingly, intentionally, and fraudulently adulterate, or cause to be adulterated, such drugs, chemicals, or medical preparations, he shall be deemed guilty of a misdemeanor, and upon conviction thereof be liable to a penalty not exceeding one hundred dollars, and in addition thereto his name shall be stricken from the register.

SEC. 2021. It shall be unlawful for any person to retail any poisons enumerated in schedules A and B, as follows, to wit:

### SCHEDULE A.

Arsenic and its preparations, corrosive sublimate, white precipitate, red precipitate, biniodide of mercury, cyanide of potassium, hydrocyanic acid, strychnia, and all other poisonous vegetable alkaloids and their salts, essential oil of bitter almonds, opium and its preparations, except paregoric and other preparations of opium containing less than two grains to the ounce.

### SCHEDULE B.

Aconite, belladonna, colchicum, conium, nux vomica, henbane, savin, ergot, cotton root, cantharides, creosote, digitalis and their pharmaceutical preparations, croton oil, chloroform, chloral hydrate, sulphate of zinc, mineral acids, carbolic acid, and oxalic acid, without distinctly labeling the bottle, box, vessel, or paper in which the said poison is contained, and also the outside wrapper or cover with the name of the article, the word "poison," and the name and place of the seller; nor shall it be lawful for any person to sell or deliver any poisons enumerated in said schedules A and B unless upon due inquiry it be found that the purchaser is aware of its poisonous character, and represents that it is to be used for a legitimate purpose. Nor shall it be lawful for any registered pharmacist to sell any poisons included in schedule A without, before delivering the same to the purchaser, causing an entry to be made in a book kept for that purpose, stating the date of sale, the name and address of the purchaser, the name and quality of the poison sold, the purpose for which it is represented by the purchaser to be required, and the name of the dispenser; such book to be always open for inspection by the proper authorities and to be preserved for reference at least five years. The provisions of this section shall not apply to the dispensing of poisons in not unusual quantities or doses upon the prescriptions of practitioners of medicine.

SEC. 2022. Nothing contained in the foregoing sections of this title shall apply to or interfere with the business of any practitioner of medicine who does not keep open shop for the retailing of medicines and poisons, nor with the business of wholesale dealers, but the preceding section and the penalties for its violation shall apply to such persons.

SEC. 2023. Any person who shall attempt to procure registration for himself or for any other person under this title by making or causing to be made any false representation shall be deemed guilty of a misdemeanor, and shall, upon conviction thereof, be liable to a penalty not exceeding five hundred dollars. Any registered pharmacist who shall permit the compounding and dispensing of prescriptions of medical practitioners in his store or place of business by any person or persons not registered, or any person not registered who shall keep open shop for the retailing or dispensing of medicines and poisons, or who shall fraudulently represent himself to be registered, or any registered pharmacist or dealer in medicines who shall fail to comply with the regulations and provisions of this title, in relation to the retailing and dispensing of poisons, shall, for every such offence, be deemed guilty of a misdemeanor, and upon conviction thereof be liable to a penalty of fifty dollars.

SEC. 2024. Each and every penalty recovered under this title shall be paid to the trustees of the College of Pharmacy, and shall form and be known as the library fund of said College of Pharmacy, and shall be expended for the purchase of books for the library of said college.

## CHAPTER 361 OF THE LAWS OF 1884.

AN ACT to establish a State board of pharmacy, and to regulate the practice of pharmacy throughout the State of New York, except in the counties of New York, Kings, and Erie.

Passed May 24, 1884; three-fifths being present.

*The people of the State of New York, represented in Senate and Assembly, do enact as follows:*

SEC. 14 (as amended by L. 1887, ch. 676). This act shall not apply to the counties of New York, Kings, and Erie: *Provided, however,* That a license as a pharmacist, granted any person after examination by any board of pharmacy legally created under the laws of this State, shall entitle said persons to a license, or a certificate of registration as a pharmacist, from any board of pharmacy legally created under the laws of this State upon presenting to such board his said license and complying with the formal requirements of said laws.

## CHAPTER 181 OF THE LAWS OF 1889.

### AN ACT relating to the practice of pharmacy.

Became a law without the approval of the governor, in accordance with the provisions of article four, section nine, of the constitution, April 24, 1889. Passed, three-fifths being present.

*The people of the State of New York, represented in Senate and Assembly, do enact as follows:*

SECTION 1. To entitle any person to a license as a pharmacist or assistant pharmacist from any board of pharmacy created under the laws of this State he must prove to the board of pharmacy to which application is made, in addition to the present requirements of the law relating to the granting of licenses by such boards, that he is a resident of the city, county, or district for which the board of pharmacy to which application is made is created, or, if a nonresident, that he intends to practice in said city, county, or district; that he has not applied for a license to, or been examined by, any other board of pharmacy of this State and been refused such license within six months immediately preceding, which proof may be made by his own affidavit.

SEC. 2. All acts and parts of acts inconsistent with the provisions of this act are hereby repealed.

SEC. 3. This act shall take effect immediately.

## THE PENAL CODE OF THE STATE OF NEW YORK.

SEC. 401. An apothecary, or druggist, or a person employed as clerk or salesman by an apothecary or druggist, or otherwise carrying on business as a dealer in drugs or medicines, who, in putting up any drugs or medicines, or making up any prescription, or filling any order for drugs or medicines, willfully, negligently, or ignorantly omits to label the same, or puts any untrue label, stamp, or other designation of contents upon any box, bottle, or other package containing a drug or medicine, or substitutes a different article for any article prescribed or ordered, or puts up a greater or less quantity of any article than that prescribed or ordered, or otherwise deviates from the terms of the prescription or order which he undertakes to follow, in consequence of which human life or health is endangered, is guilty of a misdemeanor.

SEC. 402. An apothecary, or druggist, or a person employed as clerk or salesman by an apothecary or druggist, or otherwise carrying on business as a dealer in drugs or medicines, who sells or gives any poison or poisonous substance without first recording in a book, to be kept for that purpose, the name and residence of the person receiving such poison, together with the kind and quantity of such poison received, and the name and residence of some person known to such dealer as a witness to the transaction, except upon the written order or prescription of some practicing physician whose name is attached to the order, is guilty of a misdemeanor.

SEC. 403. A person whose duty it is by the last section to keep a book for recording the sale or gift of poisons, who willfully refuses to permit any person to inspect said book upon reasonable demand, made during ordinary business hours, is punishable by a fine not exceeding fifty dollars.

SEC. 404. (As am'd by L 1886 ch. 390.) A person who sells, gives away, or disposes of any poison or poisonous substance (except upon the order or prescription of a regularly authorized practicing physician), without attaching to the vial, box, or parcel containing such poisonous substance a label with the name and residence of such person, the word "poison," and the name of such poison, all written or printed thereon in plain and legible characters; and a person who, after the first day of January, eighteen hundred and eighty-seven, sells, gives away, or disposes of, or offers for sale any sulphate or other preparation of opium or morphine, except paregoric and those preparations containing two grains or less of opium or morphine to the ounce, without attaching to the bottle, vial, box, or package containing such sulphate or other preparation of opium or morphine, a scarlet label lettered in white letters, plainly naming the contents thereof, with the name and residence of such person, is guilty of a misdemeanor.

SEC. 405. No person employed in a drug store or apothecary's shop shall prepare a medical prescription unless he has served two years' apprenticeship in such a store or shop, or is a graduate of a medical college or college of pharmacy, except under the direct supervision of some person possessing one of those qualifications; nor shall any proprietor or other person in charge of such store or shop permit any person not possessing such qualifications to prepare a medical prescription in his store or shop, except under such supervision. A person violating any provision of this section is guilty of a misdemeanor, punishable by a fine not exceeding one hundred dollars, or by imprisonment not exceeding six months; and in case of death ensuing from such violation, the person offending is guilty of a felony, punishable by a fine not less than one thousand dollars nor more than five thousand dollars, or by imprisonment not less than two years nor more than four years, or by both such fine and imprisonment.

CHAPTER 636 OF THE LAWS OF 1887.

AN ACT to regulate the sale of morphine by druggists and apothecaries in this State.

Passed June 21, 1887; three-fifths being present.

*The people of the State of New York, represented in Senate and Assembly, do enact as follows:*

SECTION 1. From and after the passage of this act no pharmacist, druggist, apothecary, or other person shall refill, more than once, prescriptions containing opium or morphine or preparations of either in which the dose of opium shall exceed one-fourth grain or morphine one-twentieth grain, except with the verbal or written order of a physician.

SEC. 2. Any person violating the provisions of section one of this act shall be deemed guilty of a misdemeanor, and shall, upon conviction thereof, be fined not less than ten dollars nor more than twenty-five dollars, in the discretion of the court, for each and every such offense.

SEC. 3. This act shall take effect immediately.

## NORTH CAROLINA.

*The General Assembly of North Carolina do enact:*

SECTION 1. That E. M. Nadal, S. J. Hinsdale, William Simpson, E. H. Meadows, T. C. Smith, John S. Pescud, and such other persons as may be associated with them under the provisions of this act, be and the same are hereby, made a body corporate under the name and style of the North Carolina Pharmaceutical Association, and by said name shall have the right to sue and be sued, to plead and be impleaded, to purchase and hold real estate and grant the same, to have and to use a common seal, and to do such other things and perform such other acts as appertain to bodies corporate and politic, not inconsistent with the constitution and laws of the State.

SEC. 2. The object of said association is to unite the pharmacists and druggists of this State for mutual aid, encouragement, and improvement; to encourage scientific research, develop pharmaceutical talent; to elevate the standard of professional thought, and ultimately restrict the practice of pharmacy to properly qualify [qualified] druggists and apothecaries.

SEC. 3. It shall be unlawful from and after the passage of this act, except as hereinafter provided, for any person, unless a registered pharmacist within the meaning of this act, to open or conduct any pharmacy or store for retailing, dispensing, or compounding medicines or poisons, or for any one not a registered pharmacist to prepare a physician's prescriptions, except under the supervision of a registered pharmaceutist, in the State of North Carolina: *Provided*, That nothing herein contained shall prevent the sale of patent or proprietary medicines, quinine, epsom salts, castor oil, essence of peppermint, paregoric, laudanum in original packages, calomel, camphor, or sweet oil.

SEC. 4. Any person, in order to be registered, shall be a graduate of some college in pharmacy recognized by the North Carolina board of pharmacy, or shall, at the passage of this act, have had three years' practical experience in the preparation of physicians' prescriptions, and in compounding and vending medicines and poisons, or shall be a licentiate of pharmacy of the board of pharmacy of North Carolina.

SEC. 5. Pharmaceutists claiming the right of registration under this act, on account of practical experience, shall, within ninety days after its passage, show to the satisfaction of the board of pharmacy to be created by this act that they have had three (3) years' practical experience in the preparation of physicians' prescriptions, and in compounding and vending medicines and poisons: *Provided*, That nothing in this section shall apply to any person or persons in business on their own account upon the passage of this act. Licentiates in pharmacy must have had three years' experience in stores where prescriptions of medical practitioners have been prepared, and shall have passed an examination before the board of pharmacy of this State. The board of pharmacy may register, without further examination, the licentiates of such other boards of pharmacy as they may deem proper.

SEC. 6. This association shall elect ten of its members—from whom the governor selects five—who shall compose the board of pharmacy. The board is empowered to transact all business relating to the legal practice of pharmacy; to examine into and adjudicate upon all cases of abuse, fraud, adulteration, substitution, or malpractice, and to enforce all the provisions of the law, and to render an annual account to the proper State authorities and to the association. Any one examined by the board shall pay a fee of five dollars. In case of failure to pass a satisfactory examination he shall be granted a second examination, without the payment of a further fee. It shall be the duty of the members of the board, after receipt of notification of their appointment, to appear before the clerk of the county in which they individually reside, and make and subscribe to an oath properly and faithfully to discharge the duties of their office; and within thirty days thereafter meet and organize by the election of a president, secretary, and treasurer of said board. The secretary and treasurer shall be elected to serve for a term of five years, and the term of office of the other members shall be determined by lot. Vacancies in the board shall be filled as required in section 12. The board shall hold meetings at least once annually or oftener, as the business of the board may require. The secretary shall give each member of the board not less than ten days' notice of each meeting. Three members shall constitute a quorum. It shall be the duty of the board to examine all persons applying for examination in proper form, and to register such as shall establish their rights to registration in accordance with the provisions of this act.

The secretary and treasurer of said board shall be a bonded officer held in bond of one thousand dollars, to be made to the said North Carolina pharmaceutical association and approved by the executive committee of said association.

SEC. 7. It shall be the duty of the secretary of the board of pharmacy to keep a book of registration at some convenient place, of which due notice shall be given through the public press, in which shall be entered, under the supervision of the board, the names and places of business of all persons coming under the provisions of this act, and a statement to be signed by the person making the application of such facts in the case as he may claim to justify his application. The fee for registration of proprietors shall not exceed two dollars, and for those in the employ of others shall not exceed one dollar. The secretary shall give receipts for all moneys received by him, which moneys shall be used for the purpose of defraying the expenses of the board of pharmacy; and any surplus shall be for the benefit of said association. The salary of the secretary shall be fixed by this board, and shall be paid out of the fees for examination and registration. Each member of the board of pharmacy shall be paid the sum of five dollars for every day during which he is engaged in the service of the board, and all necessary expenses incurred in attending the meetings of the same. It shall be the duty of the board to investigate all complaints of disregard, noncompliance, or violation of the provisions of this act, and to bring the same to the notice of the proper prosecuting officer, whenever there appears to the board reasonable grounds of complaint. The board is hereby empowered to make such rules and regulations as it shall find necessary for carrying into effect the provisions of this law, not inconsistent with the purpose and spirit of the same.

SEC. 8. Every person, from and after the passage of this act, shall be held responsible for the quality of all drugs, chemicals, and medicines he may sell or dispense, with the exception of those sold in the original packages of the manufacturers, and also those known as "patent medicines;" and should he intentionally adulterate, or cause to be adulterated, or expose to sale, knowing the same to be adulterated, such drugs, chemicals, or medical preparations, he shall be deemed guilty of a misdemeanor, and, upon conviction thereof, be liable to a penalty not exceeding one hundred dollars, and in addition thereto his name shall be stricken from the register. Every registered pharmacist who desires to continue the practice of his profession shall annually thereafter, within thirty days next preceding the annual meeting of the board of pharmacy, pay to the secretary of the said board a registration fee of one dollar, for which he shall receive a renewal of said certificate of registration. Any registered pharmacist failing to renew his registration as required by this section, and continuing in the exercise of his profession, shall be guilty of a misdemeanor.

SEC. 9. It shall be unlawful for any person under a penalty of $25 for each and every offense, from and after the passage of this act, except as provided herein, to retail any poison enumerated in schedules A and B, as follows, to wit:

SCHEDULE A.

Arsenic and its preparations, corrosive sublimate, white precipitate, red precipitate, biniodide of mercury, cyanide of potassium, hydrocyanic acid, strychnine, and essential oil of bitter almonds.

SCHEDULE B.

Aconite, belladonna, colchicum, conium, nux vomica, henbane, savin, ergot, cotton root, cantharides, creosote, digitalis, and their pharmaceutical preparations, croton oil, chloroform, chloral hydrate, sulphate of zinc, carbolic acid, oxalic acid, opium and its preparations, except paregoric and other preparations of opium containing less than two grains to the ounce, and other poisons, without distinctly labeling the bottle, box, vessel, or paper in which said poison is contained, with the name of the article, the word "poison," and a vignette representing a skull and crossbones, and the name and the place of business of the seller; nor shall it be lawful for any person to sell or deliver any poison enumerated in said schedules A and B, unless upon due inquiry it is found that the purchaser is aware of its poisonous nature, and represents that it is to be used for a legitimate purpose; nor shall it be lawful for any person to sell any poison included in schedule A without, before delivering the same to the purchaser, causing an entry to be made in a book kept for that purpose, stating the date of the sale, the name and the address of the purchaser, the name and quality of the poison sold, the purpose for which it is represented by the purchaser to be required, and the name of the dispenser—such book to be always open to proper authorities for inspection. The provisions of this section shall not apply to the dispensing of poisons in usual doses, and by physicians' prescriptions.

SEC. 10. Nothing contained in the foregoing section shall apply to or interfere with the business of any practitioner of medicine who does not keep open shop for retailing of medicines and poisons; nor with the business of wholesale dealers, excepting section 9, and the penalties of its violation.

SEC. 11. Any person who shall permit, by willful neglect, the compounding and dispensing of prescriptions in his store or place of business, by any person or persons not registered except under the supervision of a registered pharmaceutist, or any person not registered who shall keep open shop for the retailing or dispensing of medicines or poisons, or who shall fraudulently represent himself to be registered, or any registered pharmacist, or any dealer in medicines, who shall fail to comply with the regulations and provisions of this act in relation to retailing and dispensing of poison, shall, for every offense, be deemed guilty of a misdemeanor, and, upon conviction thereof, be liable to a penalty not exceeding twenty-five dollars.

SEC. 12. Immediately on passage of this act the governor shall appoint five reputable and practicing pharmacists doing business within the State, from ten of said pharmacists recommended to him by the North Carolina pharmaceutical association; said pharmacists so appointed shall constitute the board of pharmacy of the State of North Carolina, and shall hold office for the term of one, two, three, four, and five years, respectively, as herein provided, and until their successors have been duly elected and qualified. "The North Carolina pharmaceutical association shall annually thereafter elect a pharmacist from their number to fill the vacancy annually occurring in said board. Said pharmacist so elected shall be commissioned by the governor and hold office for the term of five years and until his successor has been duly elected and qualified. In case of death, resignation, or removal from the State of any member of said board of pharmacy, the said board shall elect in his place a pharmacist who is a member of said association, to serve as a member of the board for the remainder of the term."

SEC. 13. The penalties prescribed by this act shall be recovered by suits in the name of the people of this State, according to the statutes in such cases provided, to be prosecuted by the proper officers of the counties, respectively, where the violations of the provisions of this act may be committed.

SEC. 14. Any pharmacist failing to comply with the requirements of sections five and eight within ninety days from and after the passage of this act shall forfeit his right to registration, and shall appear before the board of pharmacy for examination, as provided in section five of this act.

SEC. 15. All acts or portions of acts conflicting with the provisions of this act are hereby repealed.

SEC. 16. It shall be the duty of the sheriffs of the counties to see that the provisions of this act are enforced.

SEC. 17. This act may for all purposes be quoted under the title of the "Pharmacy Act of 1881."

SEC. 18. This act shall be in force from and after the first day of June next. Ratified this 12th day of March, A. D. 1881.

[NOTE.—The provisions of the act amending sections four and five of the "Pharmacy Act," as ratified on January 27, 1891, and which went into effect July 1, 1891, only apply to towns of over 800 inhabitants.—SECRETARY.]

In explanation of the above note, it will be necessary to say that heretofore physicians had the legal right to register as pharmacists anywhere in the State; now that right has been limited to physicians resident of towns less than 800 inhabitants; all others have to pass the examination of the State board of pharmacy.

Pharmacists registered in this State are exempt from jury duty.

WM. SIMPSON,<br>Sec'y N. C. Board Pharmacy.

## NORTH DAKOTA.

AN ACT to regulate the practice of pharmacy, the licensing of persons to carry on such practice, and the sale of poisons in the State of North Dakota.

*Be it enacted by the Legislative Assembly of the State of North Dakota:*

SECTION 1. That it shall be unlawful for any person other than a registered pharmacist to retail, compound, or dispense drugs, medicines, or poisons, or to institute or conduct any pharmacy, store, or shop for retailing, compounding, or dispensing drugs, medicines, or poisons, unless such person shall be a registered pharmacist or shall employ or place in charge of said pharmacy, store, or shop a registered pharmacist within the full meaning of this act, except as hereinafter provided for.

SEC. 2. In order to be registered within the full meaning of this act, all persons must either be graduates in pharmacy or shall have been engaged in the dispensing of drugs and medicines for a period of not less than four years, in the preparation of physicians' prescriptions, or shall be licentiates in pharmacy.

*SEC. 3. Licentiates in pharmacy shall be such persons as have had two successive years' practical experience in drug stores wherein the prescriptions of medical practitioners are compounded, and have sustained a satisfactory examination before the State board of pharmacy, hereinafter mentioned. The board of pharmacy may grant certificates of registration to graduates in pharmacy who have obtained a diploma from such colleges or schools of pharmacy as shall be approved by said boards, or to licentiates or such other State or Territorial board as it may deem proper, without further examination.

---

*Sections 3, 5, 8, 10, 11, and 12 have been amended as shown by following act, approved March 6, 1893:

AN ACT to amend an act entitled "An act to regulate the practice of pharmacy, the licensing of persons to carry on such practice, and the sale of poisons in the State of North Dakota," approved March 20th, 1890.

*Be it enacted by the Legislative Assembly of the State of North Dakota:*

SECTION 1. That section 3 of said act be amended to read as follows:

"SEC. 3. Licentiates in pharmacy shall be such persons as have had four successive years' practical experience in drug stores wherein the prescriptions of medical practitioners are compounded, and have sustained a satisfactory examination before the State board of pharmacy, hereinafter mentioned. The board of pharmacy may grant certificates of registration to graduates in pharmacy who have obtained a diploma from such colleges or schools of pharmacy as shall be approved by said boards, or to licentiates or such other State or Territorial board as it may deem proper, without further examination."

SEC. 2. That section 5 of said act be amended by adding thereto the following:

"SEC. 5. The said board shall also have the power to cancel the certificate of any registered pharmacist for intemperance, incompetency, or illegal sale of intoxicating liquors, in the following manner:

SEC. 4. Upon the passage of this act the North Dakota pharmaceutical association shall select five reputable and practicing pharmacists doing business in the State, from which number the governor of the State shall appoint three. The said three pharmacists duly elected and appointed shall constitute the board of pharmacy of the State of North Dakota, and shall hold office as designated in their appointments for the term of one, two and three years, as hereinafter provided, and until their successors have been appointed and qualified. Annually thereafter the North Dakota pharmaceutical association shall select three pharmacists, who shall be members in good standing, from which number the governor of the State shall appoint one to fill the vacancy annually occurring in said board. The term of office shall be three years. In case of resignation or removal from the State of any member of said board, or of a vacancy occurring from any cause, the governor shall fill the vacancy by appointing a pharmacist from the names last submitted, to serve as a member of the board for the remainder of the term.

SEC. 5. Said board shall, within thirty days after their appointment and qualification, meet and organize by the selection of a president and secretary from the number of its own members, who shall be elected for the term of one year and shall perform the duties prescribed by the board. It shall be the duty of the board to examine all applications for registration submitted in proper form; to grant certificates of registration to such persons as may be entitled to the same under the provisions of this act; to cause the prosecution of all persons violating its provisions; to report annually to the governor, and to the North Dakota pharmaceutical association, upon the condition of pharmacy in the State, which said report shall also furnish a record of the proceedings of said board for the year, as well as the names of all pharmacists duly registered under this act. The board shall hold meetings for the examination of all applicants for registration and transaction of such other business as shall pertain to its duties at least twice, or not more than four times, a year, at the discretion of the board; and the said board shall give thirty days' public notice, in three of the pharmaceutical journals of general circulation of the State, of the time and place of such meeting. The said board shall also have power to make by-laws for the proper execution of its duties under this act, and shall keep a book

"Upon the sworn complaint of at least three reputable citizens charging any registered pharmacist with intemperance, incompetency, or illegal sale of intoxicating liquors, the board shall appoint a time and place for hearing of said charges and shall give the pharmacist so charged at least ten days' notice by mail of the time and place of said hearing, when he shall appear and answer said charges.

"If the board shall find any one or all of said charges to be true they shall forthwith cancel the certificate of said pharmacist and his registry as a pharmacist entitled to do business in North Dakota."

SEC. 3. That section 8 of said act be amended to read as follows:

"SEC. 8. Every person claiming registration as a registered pharmacist under section six of this act shall, before a certificate is granted, pay the secretary of the State board of pharmacy the sum of three dollars, and a like sum shall be paid to said secretary by such licentiates of other boards who shall apply for registration under this act; and every applicant for registration by examination shall pay to the secretary the sum of five (5) dollars before such examination be attempted: *Provided*, That in case of failure to pass a satisfactory examination, he may be reëxamined at any regular meeting of the board by paying a fee of three (3) dollars: *Provided*, That on arbitration under this act as a pharmacist entitled to membership in the North Dakota Pharmaceutical Association."

SEC. 4. That section 10 of said act be amended to read as follows:

"SEC. 10. Every registered pharmacist who desires to continue the practice of his profession shall, annually, during the time he shall continue such practice, on such date as the board of pharmacy shall determine, pay to the secretary of said board a registration fee, the amount of which shall be fixed by the board, and which in no of registration in which shall be entered the names and places of business of all persons registered under this act, which registration book shall also contain such facts as such persons claim to justify their registration. Two members of said board shall constitute a quorum.

SEC. 6. Every person claiming the right of registration under this act who shall, within three months after the passage of this act and the organization of this board, forward to the board of pharmacy satisfactory proof supported by his affidavit that he was engaged in the business of dispensing pharmacist on his own account in the State of North Dakota at the time of the passage of this act as provided in section two (2) shall, upon the payment of the fee hereinafter mentioned, be granted a certificate of registration: *Provided*, That in case of failure or neglect to register as herein specified, then such person shall, in order to be registered, comply with the requirements provided for registration as licentiates in pharmacy within the meaning of this act.

SEC. 7. That the foregoing provisions of this act shall not apply to or affect any person having four consecutive years' experience in the dispensing of and compounding of prescriptions of regular practitioners, and employed as a pharmacist of North Dakota at the passage of this act, only in so far as relates to registration and fees hereinafter provided for.

*SEC. 8. Every person claiming registration as a registered pharmacist under section six of this act shall, before a certificate is granted, pay to the secretary of the State board of pharmacy the sum of two (2) dollars, and a like sum shall be paid to said secretary by such licentiates of other boards who shall apply for registration under this act; and every applicant for registration by examination shall pay to the said secretary the sum of five (5) dollars before such examination be attempted: *Provided*, That in case of failure to pass a satisfactory examination he may be reëxamined at any regular meeting of the board by paying a fee of three (3) dollars.

SEC. 9. Any assistant or clerk in pharmacy who shall not have the qualifications of a registered pharmacist within the meaning of this act, not less than eighteen years of age, who shall have been employed or engaged two years or more in drug stores where the prescriptions of medical practitioners are compounded, and shall furnish satisfactory evidence to that effect to the State board of pharmacy, shall,

case shall exceed three (3) dollars, in return for which payment he shall receive a renewal of said registration and renewal of membership in the North Dakota pharmaceutical association.

"Every certificate of registration and every renewal of such certificate shall be conspicuously exposed in a pharmacy to which it applies. It shall be the duty of every registered pharmacist, or assistant pharmacist, upon changing his place of business to notify, by letter, within thirty days, the secretary of the State board of pharmacy of such change, and to enclose a fee of fifty cents, upon receipt of which the secretary shall make the necessary alterations.

If not notified within the time specified, the name of such registered pharmacist or assistant pharmacist shall be stricken from the register. The secretary shall publish annually a list of all persons who are duly registered as "registered pharmacist" and "assistant pharmacist" in the State, and a copy shall be mailed to each "registered pharmacist" and "assistant pharmacist" in the State.

SEC. 5. That section 11 of said act shall be amended to read as follows:

SEC. 11. The secretary of the State board of pharmacy shall receive a salary which shall be determined by said board. He shall also receive his traveling and other expenses incurred in the performance of his official duty. The other members of said board shall receive the sum of five (5) dollars for each day actually engaged in such service, and all legitimate and necessary expenses incurred in attending the meeting of the said board, or while performing strictly official duties. Said expenses shall be paid from the fees and penalties received by said board under the provisions of this act, and no part of the salary or other expenses of said board shall be paid upon making application for registration, and upon payment to the secretary of the said board of a fee of one (1) dollar, be entitled to a certificate as a "registered assistant," which said certificate shall entitle him to continue in such duties as clerk or assistant; but such certificate shall not entitle him to engage in business on his own account, unless he shall have had at least four years' practical experience in pharmacy at the time of the passage of this act. Annually thereafter, during the time he shall continue in such duties, he shall pay to said secretary a sum not to exceed fifty (50) cents, for which he shall receive a renewal of his certificate.

\* SEC. 10. Every registered pharmacist who desires to continue the practice of his profession shall, annually, during the time he shall continue such practice, on such date as the board of pharmacy shall determine, pay to the secretary of said board a registration fee, the amount of which shall be fixed by the board, and which in no case shall exceed two (2) dollars, in return for which payment he shall receive a renewal of said registration. Every certificate of registration and every renewal of such certificate shall be conspicuously exposed in the pharmacy to which it applies. It shall be the duty of every registered pharmacist or assistant pharmacist, upon changing his place of business, to notify by letter, within thirty days, the secretary of the State board of pharmacy of such change, and to inclose a fee of fifty cents, upon receipt of which the secretary shall make the necessary alterations. If not notified within the time specified, the name of such registered pharmacist or assistant pharmacist shall be stricken from the register. The secretary shall publish annually a list of all persons who are duly registered as "registered pharmacists" and "assistant pharmacists," a copy of which shall be mailed free to each "registered pharmacist" and "assistant pharmacist" in the State.

\* SEC. 11. The secretary of the State board of pharmacy shall receive a salary, which shall be determined by said board; he shall also receive his traveling and other expenses incurred in the performance of his official duties. The other members of said board shall receive the sum of five (5) dollars for each day actually engaged in such service and all legitimate and necessary expenses incurred in attending the meeting of said board, or while performing strictly official duties. Said expenses shall be paid from the fees and penalties received by said board under the provisions of this act, and no part of the salary or other expenses of said board shall be paid out of the public treasury. All moneys received by said board in excess of said allowances and other expenses hereinbefore provided for shall be held by the secretary of said board as a special fund for meeting the expenses of said board, said secretary giving such bonds as the said board shall from time to time direct and approve. The said board shall, in its annual report to the governor, and to the North Dakota pharmaceutical association, render an account of all moneys received and disbursed by them pursuant to this act.

---

out of the public treasury. All moneys received by said board in excess of said allowance and other expenses, hereinbefore provided for, shall be held by the treasurer of said board as a special fund for meeting the expenses of said board and the expenses of this annual meeting and report of this North Dakota pharmaceutical association and other necessary expenses which may be incurred by said association, said treasurer giving such bonds as the said board shall from time to time direct and approve. The said board shall, in its annual report to the governor and to the North Dakota pharmaceutical association, render an account of all moneys received and disbursed by them pursuant to this act.

SEC. 6. That section 12 of said act shall be amended to read as follows:

SEC. 12. Any person not being or having in his employ a registered pharmacist within the full meaning of this (act) who shall retail, compound, or compense [dispense] medicines, or who shall take, use, or exhibit the title of a registered pharmacist, or announce or advertise in any manner that would lead the public to believe that he was a registered pharmacist, shall be deemed guilty of a misdemeanor, and, upon conviction shall, for each and every offense, be liable to a penalty not to exceed fifty (50) dollars. Any registered pharmacist or other person who shall permit the com-

*SEC. 12. Any person not being or not having in his employ a registered pharmacist within the full meaning of this [act], who shall retail, compound, or dispense medicines, or who shall take, use, or exhibit the title of a registered pharmacist shall be deemed guilty of a misdemeanor, and upon conviction shall, for each and every offense, be liable to a penalty not to exceed fifty (50) dollars. Any registered pharmacist or other person who shall permit the compounding and dispensing of prescriptions or the vending of drugs, medicines, or poisons in his store or place of business except under the supervision of a registered pharmacist, or any pharmacist who, while continuing business, shall fail or neglect to procure his annual registration, or any person who shall willfully make any false representation to procure registration for himself or any other person, or who shall violate any other provision of this act shall be deemed guilty of a misdemeanor, and upon conviction shall, for each and every offense, be liable to a penalty not to exceed fifty (50) dollars: *Provided*, That nothing in this act shall in any manner interfere with the business of any physician in regular practice, nor prevent him from supplying his patients with such articles as may seem to him proper, nor prevent him from receiving a certificate as a registered pharmacist upon his producing a statement from the North Dakota board of medical examiners that he has answered at least 70 per cent of the questions asked at their examination in chemistry, pharmacy, and materia medica: *Provided, further*, That physicians registered on account of residence in the State be registered as "registered pharmacists" on presentation of their certificate from the North Dakota medical board; nor with the making of proprietary medicines or medicines placed in sealed packages with the name of the contents and the pharmacist or physician by whom prepared or compounded; nor prevent shopkeepers from dealing in and selling the commonly-used medicines and poisons, if such medicines are put up by a registered pharmacist, or from dealing in and selling of patent or proprietary medicines, nor with the exclusive wholesale business of any dealers.

SEC. 13. Every proprietor or conductor of a drug store shall be held responsible for the quality of all drugs, chemicals, and medicines sold or dispensed by him except those sold in the original packages of the manufacturer and except those articles or preparations known as patent or proprietary medicines. Any person who shall knowingly, willfully, or fraudulently falsify or adulterate, or cause to be falsified or adulterated, any drug or medical substance, or any preparation authorized or recognized by any standard work on pharmacy, or used or intended to be used in medical practice, or shall mix or cause to be mixed with any such drug or medicinal substance any foreign or inert substance whatsoever for the purpose of destroying or weakening its medicinal power and effect, or of lessening its cost, and shall willfully, knowingly, or fraudulently sell, or cause the same to be sold for medicinal

---

pounding and dispensing of prescriptions or the vending of drugs, medicines, or poisons in his store or place of business except under the supervision of a registered pharmacist, or any pharmacist who, while continuing business, shall fail or neglect to procure his annual registration, or any person who shall wilfully make any false representation to procure registration for himself or any other person, or who shall violate any other provision of this act shall be deemed guilty of a misdemeanor, and, upon conviction shall, for each and every offense, be liable to a penalty not to exceed fifty (50) dollars: *Provided*, That nothing in this act shall in any manner interfere with the business of any physician in regular practice, nor prevent him from supplying his patients with such articles as may seem proper, nor with the making of proprietary medicines or medicines placed in sealed packages with the name of the contents and the pharmacist or physician by whom prepared or compounded; nor prevent shopkeepers from dealing in and selling the commonly used medicines and poisons, if such medicines are put up by a registered pharmacist, or from dealing in and selling patent or proprietary medicines, nor with the exclusive wholesale business of any dealers.

Approved, March 6, 1893.

purposes, shall be deemed guilty of a misdemeanor, and upon conviction thereof shall pay a penalty not exceeding five hundred (500) dollars, and shall forfeit to the State of North Dakota all articles so adulterated.

SEC. 14. It shall be deemed unlawful for any person to retail any poisons enumerated in schedules A and B, except as hereinafter provided for.

### SCHEDULE A.

Arsenic and its preparations, corrosive sublimate, white precipitate, red precipitate, biniodide of mercury, cyanide of potassium, hydrocyanic acid, strychnia, and all other poisons, vegetable alkaloids and their salts, essential oil of bitter almonds, opium and its preparations, except paregoric and other preparations of opium with less than two grains to the ounce.

### SCHEDULE B.

Aconite, belladonna, colchicum, conium, nux vomica, henbane, savin, ergot, cotton root, cantharides, creosote, digitalis and their pharmaceutical preparations, croton oil, chloroform, chloral hydrate, sulphate of zinc, mineral acids, carbolic acid, and any oxalic acid.

A poison in the meaning of this act shall be any drug, chemical, or preparation which, according to standard works on medicine or materia medica, is liable to be destructive to adult human life in quantities of sixty (60) grains or less. No person shall sell at retail any poisons mentioned in schedules A and B above mentioned without affixing to the bottle, box, vessel, or package containing them the name of the contents, the word "poison," and the name and place of business of the seller, nor shall he deliver said poison to any person without satisfying himself that such poison is to be used for legitimate purposes: *Provided*, That nothing herein contained shall apply to the dispensing of physicians' prescriptions specifying poison. It shall also be the duty of such vendor of poisons, before delivering the same to the purchaser, to cause an entry to be made in a book kept for that purpose, stating the date of sale, the name and address of the purchaser, the name and quality of the poison sold, and the name of the dispenser, such book to be always kept open for inspection by the proper authorities, and to be preserved for reference for at least five years. Any person failing to comply with the requirements of this section shall be deemed guilty of a misdemeanor and shall, upon conviction, be liable to a fine of not less than five (5) dollars for each and every such omission.

SEC. 15. All suits for the recovery of the several penalties and costs prescribed in this act shall be prosecuted in the name of the State of North Dakota in any court having jurisdiction, and it shall be the duty of the State's attorney of the county wherein such offense is committed to prosecute all persons violating the provisions of this act upon proper complaint being made. All penalties collected under the provisions of this act shall inure to the board of pharmacy for the expenses and costs of the proper execution of the law.

SEC. 16. All acts or parts of acts regulating the practice of pharmacy or adulterations of drugs within this State, enacted prior to the passage of this act, which in anywise conflict with the provisions of this act, are hereby repealed: *Provided*, That nothing in this act shall be so construed as to prevent any person who has once been a member by examination and may have forfeited his membership by nonpayment of fines or fees, from renewing his registration within two years, by paying the required dues or fees, without examination.

SEC. 17. Whereas the existing laws do not provide any punishment for the violation of the provisions of the law now governing the practice of pharmacy, nor is there any schedule of poisons specified therein, thereby not only exposing the public to the danger arising from the acts of incompetent persons, but there is an existing confusion as to what drug, chemical, or preparation is termed a poison and dangerous to life, hence an emergency exists; therefore this act shall take effect and be in force from and after its passage and approval.

Approved March 20, 1890.

# OKLAHOMA.

## Chapter LXI.—Pharmacy.

AN ACT to regulate the practice of pharmacy in the Territory of Oklahoma and providing penalties for the violation of the same.

[Took effect December 25, 1890; amended March 14, 1893.]

*Be it enacted by the Legislative Assembly of the Territory of Oklahoma:*

(3624) SECTION 1. That it shall be unlawful for any person, unless a qualified pharmacist within the meaning of this act, to open or conduct any pharmacy, or for any one not a qualified pharmacist to prepare physicians' prescriptions or compound medicines except under direct supervision of a qualified pharmacist, as hereinafter provided.

(3625) SEC. 2. Any person, in order to be qualified, shall be twenty-one years old, and shall have passed a satisfactory examination before the board of pharmacy of Oklahoma Territory, or shall be a graduate in pharmacy as hereinafter provided.*

(3626) SEC. 3. Graduates in pharmacy within the meaning of this act shall be such as have obtained a diploma from a recognized college of pharmacy.

(3627) SEC. 4. Assistants in pharmacy must be eighteen years old, and have had two years' experience in stores where prescriptions of medical practitioners have been prepared, and shall have passed a satisfactory examination before the board of pharmacy of Oklahoma Territory.

(3628) SEC. 5. Within thirty days after the approval of this act the governor shall appoint a board of pharmaceutical examiners, who shall hold their offices for one, two, and three years, respectively, which appointments shall be in writing and signed by the governor and secretary of the Territory, and delivered to the persons appointed. Said board of pharmacy shall be composed of three qualified pharmacists, who are residents of the Territory, no two of whom shall be residents of the same county, and who shall have had at least five years' experience in the actual practice of pharmacy, which three are to be selected from ten names recommended by the Oklahoma pharmaceutical association. If a vacancy occur in said board, another shall be appointed as aforesaid to fill the unexpired term. At the expiration of each term of office of a member, the governor shall appoint his successor, who shall hold his office for three years. Said board shall have power to make by-laws and all necessary regulations consistent with the provisions of this act, for the proper fulfillment of their duties.*

(3629) SEC. 6. The board shall meet four times a year, to wit, on the first Tuesday in the months of January, April, July, and October. The board shall organize by electing a president, secretary, and treasurer, who shall hold their respective offices for one year, and until their successors are elected. The duties of said board shall be to examine all applicants for registration and to direct the registration, by the secretary of all persons properly qualified or entitled thereto.*

(3630) SEC. 7. The members of the board of pharmacy shall receive as compensation for their services five dollars a day and necessary expenses for each day actually employed at meetings of said board, to be paid out of the Territorial treasury: *Provided*, Such compensation and expenses shall at each meeting of the board not exceed the amount received by said board for examinations and certificates at such meeting.

(3631) SEC. 8. It shall be the duty of the secretary of the board of pharmacy to keep a book in which shall be entered under the supervision of the board of pharmacy the name and place of business of every person who shall apply for registration, and a statement signed by the person making the application of such facts as he or she may claim to justify his or her application. It shall also be the duty of the secretary to duly note the fact against the name of any qualified pharmacist who may have died, or removed from the Territory, or disposed of or relinquished

---

* Act March 14, 1893.

his business; a copy of which book, corrected quarterly, shall, by the secretary of such board, be placed on file in the office of the secretary of the Territory, and certified copies of the record so filed, certified by the secretary of the Territory, shall be evidence in all criminal prosecutions under this act and of equal force with the original. Registered pharmacists who have voluntarily retired from business for a period not exceeding one year shall not forfeit their registration: *Provided*, They shall comply with section 17 of said [this] chapter.\*

(3632) SEC. 9. Any person in order to become a qualified pharmacist within the meaning of this act, shall apply and appear for examination and registration, and shall pay to the board of pharmacy five dollars, which shall be turned into the Territorial treasury, and on passing the examination required, shall be furnished free of cost a certificate of registration, signed by said board. Should said person fail to pass a satisfactory examination, he may at any other one meeting of the board of pharmacy within twelve months, be permitted to be examined without cost.

(3633) SEC. 10. Graduates as specified in section three, shall apply for registration, and if they produce satisfactory evidence to the board of pharmacy that they have a right to be registered, shall, upon paying the said board three dollars, be furnished a certificate of registration without examination.

(3634) SEC. 11. That the provisions of this act shall not prevent any person from engaging in the business herein described as proprietor or owner thereof: *Provided*, Such proprietor or owner shall have employed in his business some registered pharmacist to fill prescriptions and compound drugs.\*

(3635) SEC. 12. Any person receiving a certificate of registration shall place it in a conspicuous place in his place of business; failing to do this, the board of pharmacy shall cancel his registration and deprive him of his certificate.

(3636) SEC. 13. Any person who continues to propound [compound] prescriptions or retail medicines without complying with this act, shall upon conviction thereof be sentenced to pay a fine of not less than fifty dollars nor more than one hundred dollars, and upon the second and every subsequent conviction, shall be sentenced to a fine of not less than one hundred dollars nor more than two hundred dollars and imprisonment for ninety days in [the] county jail.

(3637) SEC. 14. Any person who shall procure registration for himself or for another under this act by making or causing to be made any false representation, shall be guilty of a misdemeanor, and shall be fined not less than twenty-five nor more than one hundred dollars, and the name of the person so fraudulently registered shall be stricken from the register.

(3638) SEC. 15. That the board of pharmacy be, and they are hereby, authorized to institute and maintain suits and prosecutions, under the provisions of said chapter and this act, in the name of the Territory of Oklahoma.\*

(3639) SEC. 16. All courts having jurisdiction in criminal causes are required to give this act in charge to each grand jury impanelled in such courts.

(3640) SEC. 17. It shall be the duty of every registered pharmacist or assistant pharmacist, upon changing his place of business from one town to another forthwith to notify by letter the secretary of the board of pharmacy of such change, and to enclose a fee of fifty cents, upon receipt of which the secretary shall make the necessary alteration on his register. It shall also be the duty of every registered pharmacist or assistant pharmacist to notify by letter said secretary, on the first day of July in each year, whether he still continues practicing pharmacy at registered place of business. The secretary shall notify every person who shall not have notified the board as herein provided, and in case an answer enclosing a fee of fifty cents shall not be received by the secretary within thirty days, such name shall be stricken from the register: *Provided, always*, That his name may be restored to register on the payment to the secretary within one year of a fee of five dollars. It shall

---

\* Act March 14, 1893.

be the duty of the secretary of the board to erase from the register the name of registered pharmacists who may have died, removed from or ceased to do business in this Territory, and to make all the necessary alterations in the locations of the persons registered under this act; he shall publish annually a list of all persons that are registered as pharmacist and assistant pharmacist, a copy of which shall be mailed free to each and every registered pharmacist and assistant pharmacist in the Territory.

(3641) SEC. 18. No one who habitually uses intoxicating liquors as a beverage shall be appointed on the board of pharmacy nor be licensed as a pharmacist or assistant pharmacist. The examining board shall in all cases require each applicant to file his written declaration, duly sworn to, to the effect that he does not habitually use vinous, malt, or alcoholic liquors as a beverage, and that he has not since January first, 1891, been engaged in the business of selling liquors in the Territory of Oklahoma. If said affidavit be filed after January first, 1893, the applicant shall then swear that he has not been engaged in the business of selling intoxicating liquors in the Territory of Oklahoma within the two years last past, and that he does not use intoxicants as before stated. Anyone swearing falsely in the affidavit so filed shall be guilty of perjury.

(3642) SEC. 19. It shall be unlawful for any person, from and after the passage of this act, to retail any of the following poisons, except as follows: Arsenic and its preparations, corrosive sublimate, white precipitate, red precipitate, biniodide of mercury, cyanide of potassium, hydrocyanic acid, strychnine and all other poisonous vegetable alkaloids and their salts, essential oil of bitter almonds, opium and its preparations except paregoric and other preparations of opium containing less than two grains to the ounce, aconite, belladonna, colchium, conium, nux vomica, henbane, savin, ergot, cotton root, cantharides, creosote, digitalis and their pharmaceutical preparations, croton oil, chloroform, chloral hydrate, sulphate of zinc, mineral acids, carbolic acid, and oxalic acid, without distinctly labeling the box, vessel, or paper in which the said poison is contained, and also the outside wrapper or cover, with the name of the article, the word "poison," and the name and place of business of the seller. Nor shall it be lawful for any registered pharmacist to sell any of the poisons above enumerated without, before delivering the same to the purchaser, causing an entry to be made in a book kept for that purpose, stating the date of sale, the name and address of the purchaser, the name of the poison sold, the purpose for which it is represented by the purchaser to be required, and the name of the dispenser, such book to be always open for inspection by the proper authorities, and to be preserved for at least five years. The provisions of this section shall not apply to the dispensing of poisons in not unusual quantities or doses, upon the prescriptions of practitioners of medicine. Any violation of the provisions of this section shall make the offender liable for a fine of not less than twenty-five dollars and not more than one hundred dollars, and upon conviction for the second offense, in addition to the fine, he shall have his name stricken from the register.*

(3643) SEC. 20. Any itinerant vendor of any drug, nostrum, ointment, or appliance of any kind, intended for the treatment of diseases or injury, who shall, by writing or printing, or any other method, publicly profess to cure or treat diseases, or injury, or deformity, by any drug, nostrum, or manipulation, or other expedient, shall pay a license of one hundred dollars for the term of one year or less, to be paid to the treasurer of the board of pharmacy and by him paid into the Territorial treasury, whereupon the secretary of the board shall issue a license for one year. Any person violating this section shall be deemed guilty of a misdemeanor, and shall, upon conviction, be fined in any sum not less than one hundred nor more than two hundred dollars.*

(3644) SEC. 21. That all laws and parts of laws in conflict with this act be, and the same are hereby, repealed, and that this act shall take effect and be in force from and after its passage.

*Act March 14, 1893.

STATUTES OF OKLAHOMA, CHAPTER XXV, SECTION 409, PAGE 118.

Every person who adulterates or dilutes any articles of food, drink, drug, medicine, strong, spirituous, or malt liquor, wine, or any article useful in compounding either of them, whether useful for mankind or for animals, with a fraudulent intent to offer the same, or cause or permit it to be offered for sale as unadulterated or undiluted, and every person who fraudulently sells or keeps, or offers it for sale the same as unadulterated or undiluted, knowing it to have been adulterated or diluted, is guilty of a misdemeanor.

## OREGON.

AN ACT to regulate the practice of pharmacy and the sale of poisons in the State of Oregon.

*Be it enacted by the Legislative Assembly of the State of Oregon:*

SECTION 1. That from and after the passage of this act it shall be unlawful for any person not a registered pharmacist within the meaning of this act, to conduct any pharmacy, drug store, apothecary shop, or store for the purpose of retailing, compounding, or dispensing medicines or poisons, or for the proprietor of any store or pharmacy to allow any person, except a registered pharmacist, to compound or dispense the prescriptions of physicians, or to retail or dispense poisons for medical use, except as an aid to and under the supervision of a registered pharmacist or registered physician.

SEC. 2. That within sixty days after the passage of this act the governor shall appoint five persons from among competent pharmacists of the State, who shall constitute the Oregon board of pharmacy. It shall be the duty of each member of said board, before entering upon the discharge of his duties, to appear before an officer duly authorized to administer oaths in this State, and make such oath to faithfully and impartially discharge the duties of a member of the board. The first term of said members of the board of pharmacy shall be one, two, three, four, and five years, respectively, and shall be designated by the governor in his appointments. Members of the board shall meet at such time and place as may be agreed upon, and shall proceed to first elect by ballot a president, treasurer, and secretary, who shall hold their offices for the term of one year, or until their successors are elected and qualified. Thereafter the board shall meet and hold examinations as hereinafter provided at least quarterly during each year, and any three members of the board shall constitute a quorum. The board shall have power to make such by-laws as it may deem necessary and not inconsistent with the constitution of this State or with the provisions of this act, and prescribe the qualifications of a pharmacist of this State. In case of a vacancy occurring in the board from any cause, the governor shall fill the vacancy by appointment from competent pharmacists of this State.

SEC. 3. That the secretary of the board shall receive a salary which shall be fixed by the board; he shall also receive his traveling and other expenses incurred in the performance of his official duties. The other members of the board shall receive the sum of five dollars for each day actually engaged in this service, and all legitimate and necessary expenses incurred in attending the meetings of said board. Said expenses shall be paid from the fees received by the board under the provisions of this act, and no part of the salary or other expenses of the board shall be paid out of the State treasury. All moneys received in excess of said expenses shall be held by the board as a special fund for meeting further expenses. The board shall render an annual report of the work it has accomplished to the governor, and render an account of all moneys received and disbursed by them pursuant to this act.

SEC. 4. That said board of pharmacy shall, upon application, and at such time and place and in such manner as they may determine, examine each and every person who shall desire to become registered as a registered pharmacist in this State, and if the majority of said board shall be satisfied that said person possesses the qualifications prescribed by the by-laws of said association they shall issue the proper certificate to such applicant, said certificate to be signed by not less than three members. The board of pharmacy shall be entitled to demand and receive of each person whom they examine for registration as a registered pharmacist the sum of five dollars, which shall be in full for all services; and in case the examination of such person shall prove defective and unsatisfactory, and his name be not registered, he shall be permitted to again present himself for examination, and if such examination is had within any period not exceeding twelve months thereafter no charge shall be made for the same.

SEC. 5. That any person shall be entitled to be registered as a registered pharmacist who shall be either a graduate in pharmacy, a licentiate in pharmacy, or who shall at the time this act takes effect be engaged in the business of a dispensing pharmacist in the State of Oregon, in the preparation of physicians' prescriptions, and in the vending and compounding of drugs, medicines, and poisons.

SEC. 6. That graduates in pharmacy must be such persons as have obtained a satisfactory diploma from a regularly incorporated college or school of pharmacy. Licentiates in pharmacy must be such persons as have passed a satisfactory examination before the State board of pharmacy. The said board may grant certificates of registration without further examination to the licentiates of such other boards in pharmacy as it may deem proper.

SEC. 7. Any assistant or clerk in pharmacy not having the qualification of a registered pharmacist within the meaning of this act, not less than eighteen years of age, who, at the time this act takes effect, shall have been employed or engaged two years or more in the drug stores where the prescriptions of medical practitioners are compounded, and have furnished satisfactory evidence to that effect to the State board of pharmacy, shall, upon making application for registration and upon the payment to the secretary of said board a fee of one dollar within sixty days after this act takes effect, be entitled to a certificate as a registered assistant, which said certificate shall entitle him to continue in such duties as a clerk or assistant, but shall not entitle him to assume the duties of a registered pharmacist, unless he shall subsequently become registered as a registered pharmacist, as provided in this act.

SEC. 8. Every person resident in the State of Oregon, claiming the right of registration under this act, who shall, within three months after the passage of this act, forward to the board of pharmacy satisfactory proof, supported by his affidavit, that he was engaged in the business of a dispensing pharmacist in the State of Oregon at the time of the passage of this act, or is otherwise entitled to registration as provided in this act, shall, upon payment of a fee of two dollars, be granted a certificate of registration: *Provided, however,* That in case of failure or neglect on the part of any such person or persons to apply for the registration within three months after the passage of this act, and after they shall have been duly notified by said board of pharmacy of the State of Oregon, they shall undergo an examination as provided for in section 4 of this act. Every certificate and every renewal shall be conspicuously exposed in the pharmacy to which it applies.

SEC. 9. That every registered pharmacist, apothecary, and owner of any store shall be held responsible for the quality of all drugs, chemicals, or poisons he may sell or dispose of, with the exception of those sold in original packages of the manufacturer, and also those known as proprietary and patent medicines, and [should] he knowingly intermingle and fraudulently adulterate, or cause to be adulterated, or knowingly substitute in a physician's prescription, any drug, chemicals, or medical preparations, he shall be deemed guilty of a misdemeanor, and upon conviction thereof be liable to a penalty not exceeding one hundred dollars, and in addition thereto his name shall be stricken from the register.

SEC. 10. That it shall be unlawful for any person, from and after the passage of this act, to retail any poisons commonly recognized as such without labeling the box, vessel, or paper in which said poison is contained with the name of the article, the word "poison," and the name and place of business of the seller. Nor shall it be lawful for any person to deliver or sell any poisons unless upon due inquiry it be found the purchaser is aware of its poisonous character and represents that it is to be used for a legitimate purpose. The proprietor of every drug store shall keep in his place of business a registry book in which shall be entered an accurate record of the sales of all such poisons. Any violation of this section shall make the principal of said store liable to a fine of not less than ten dollars and not more than one hundred dollars for each offense: *Provided, however*, That this section shall not apply to manufacturers making and selling at wholesale any poisons, but, provided that each box, vessel, or paper in which said poison is contained shall be labeled as above specified.

SEC. 11. Any person not being a registered pharmacist, or who shall not have complied with all the provisions of this act, who shall take, exhibit, or use the title of pharmacist, or who proposes to or does compound or dispense prescriptions of medical practitioners, or retail medicines or poisons to be used as medicines, or has not in any way followed the provisions of this act, shall be subject to indictment for each offense, and upon conviction shall be fined for the first offense fifty dollars and the cost of prosecution, and for each subsequent violation he shall be fined one hundred dollars and the cost of prosecution: *Provided*, That nothing in this act shall be construed to apply to the business of a licensed practitioner of medicines, nor to prevent such practitioner from supplying his patients with such articles as he may deem proper, nor to those who sell medicines, nor to those who sell medicines or poisons by whole sale only, nor to the manufacture or sale of proprietary or patent medicines, nor prevent shopkeepers from dealing in and selling the commonly used medicines and poisons, if such poisons and medicines are properly labeled.

SEC. 12. That any person who shall procure or attempt to procure registration for himself or for another under this act, by making or causing to be made false representations, shall be deemed guilty of a misdemeanor, and shall, upon conviction thereof, be liable to a penalty of not less than twenty-five dollars nor more than one hundred dollars, and the name of the person so falsely registered shall be stricken from the register.

## OHIO.

SECTION 1. *Be it enacted by the General Assembly of the State of Ohio*, That sections forty-four hundred and five, forty-four hundred and six, forty-four hundred and seven, forty-four hundred and eight, forty-four hundred and nine, forty-four hundred and ten, forty-four hundred and eleven, [and] forty-four hundred and twelve of the Revised Statutes of Ohio be so amended as to read as follows:

SEC. 4405. It shall be unlawful for any person not a registered pharmacist to open or conduct any pharmacy or any retail drug or chemical store as proprietor thereof unless he shall have in his employ and place, in charge of such pharmacy or store, a registered pharmacist, within the meaning of this chapter, who shall have the supervision and management of that part of the business requiring pharmaceutical skill and knowledge; or to engage in the occupation of compounding or dispensing medicines or prescriptions of physicians, or of selling at retail for medical purposes any drugs, chemicals, poisons, or pharmaceutical preparations within this State until he has complied with the provisions of this chapter: *Provided*, Nothing in this section shall apply to or in any manner interfere with the business of any physician, or prevent him supplying to his patients such articles as may seem to him proper, or to the making, or vending of patent or proprietary medicines by any retail dealer, or with the selling by any country store of copperas, borax, blue vitriol, saltpeter, sulphur, brimstone, licorice, sage, juniper berries, senna leaves, castor oil, sweet oil, spirits of turpentine, glycerin, Glauber's salt, Epsom salt, cream of tartar, bicarbonate of sodium, and of paregoric, essence of peppermint, essence of cinnamon, essence of ginger, lime syrup, syrup of ipecac, tincture of arnica, syrup of tolu, syrup of squills, spirits of camphor, number six, sweet spirits of niter, compound cathartic pills, quinine pills, and other similar preparations when compounded by a registered pharmacist, and put up in bottles and boxes bearing the label of such pharmacist or wholesale druggist, with the name of the article and directions for its use on each bottle or box, or with the exclusive wholesale business of any dealer.

SEC. 4406. The Ohio State pharmaceutical association shall immediately upon the passage of this act submit to the governor the names of ten persons, resident of this State, who have had at least ten years' experience as pharmacists and druggists, and from the names so submitted to him, or others, the governor shall, with the approval of the senate, select and appoint five persons, who shall constitute a board to be styled the Ohio board of pharmacy, and any member of the board may be removed by the governor for good cause shown him. One member of said board shall be appointed and hold his office for one year, one for two years, one for three years, one for four years, and one for five years, and until his successor shall be appointed and qualified; and at its regular annual meeting, in each and every meeting thereafter, the said Ohio State pharmaceutical association shall select and submit to the governor the names of five persons with the qualifications hereinbefore mentioned, and the governor shall, with the approval of the senate, select from the names so submitted, or others, one member of said board who shall hold his office for five years, or until his successor shall be appointed and qualified.

Any vacancy that may occur in said board shall be filled for the unexpired term by the governor, with the approval of the senate. Each member of said board shall, within ten days after his appointment, take and subscribe an oath of affirmation before a competent officer to faithfully and imparti lly perform the duties of his office.

SEC. 4407. The Ohio board of pharmacy shall hold thre regular meetings in each year, one at Cincinnati on the second Monday of Januar , one at Columbus on the second Monday of May, and one at Cleveland on the second Monday of October, and such additional meetings at such times and places as may be determined upon by said board, at each of which meetings it shall transact such business as is required of it by law; said board shall make such rules, by-laws, and regulations as may be necessary for the proper discharge of their duties, and shall make a report of its proceedings, including an itemized account of all moneys received and expended by said board, pursuant to this chapter, and a list of the names of all pharmacists duly registered under this act, to the secretary of State on the 15th of November, 1884, and annually thereafter, and to the Ohio State pharmaceutical association. Said board shall keep a book of registration open at some place in Columbus, of which due notice shall be given in three or more newspapers of general circulation in this State, in which the name and place of business of every person duly qualified under this chapter to conduct or engage in the business mentioned and described in section forty-four hundred and five shall be registered. Every person now conducting or engaged in such business in this State as proprietor or manager of the same, or who, being of the age of eighteen years, has been employed or engaged for three years preceding the passage of this act as an assistant in any retail drug store in the United States, in the compounding or dispensing of medicines on the prescriptions of physicians, who shall furnish satisfactory evidence, in writing and under oath, of such facts within three months after the publication of said notice, shall be registered as a pharmacist or assistant pharmacist, as the case may be, without examination. Every person, who shall hereafter desire to conduct or engage in such business in this State, shall appear before said board and be registered within ten days after receiving a certificate of competency and qualification from said board. The said board shall demand and receive for such registration, from each and every person registered as a pharmacist, a fee of not exceeding three dollars, and from each and every person registered as an assistant pharmacist a fee not exceeding two dollars, to be applied to the payment of the expenses arising under the provisions of this chapter: *Provided, however,* That no such fee shall be demanded of any person who has heretofore been registered as the proprietor or manager of such business, or as an assistant therein, under the provisions of any law heretofore in force in this State. Every registered pharmacist or assistant pharmacist, who desires to continue the practice of his profession, shall triennially thereafter, during the time he shall continue in such practice, on such date as said board may determine, pay to the secretary of said board a registration fee to be fixed by said board, but which shall in no case exceed, if a pharmacist, one dollar, if assistant pharmacist, fifty cents, for which he shall receive a renewal of such registration. Every certificate of registration granted under this act shall be conspicuously exposed in the prescription department of the drug or chemical store to which it applies, or in which the assistant is engaged. The secretary of said board shall receive a salary which shall be fixed by said board ; he shall also receive his traveling and other expenses incurred in the performance of his official duties. The other members of said board shall receive the sum of three dollars for each day actually engaged in the service thereof and all legitimate and necessary expenses incurred in attending the meetings of said board. Said salary per diem and expenses shall be paid after an itemized statement of the same has been rendered and approved by the board from the fees and penalties received by said board under the provisions of this act. All moneys received in excess of said per diem allowance and other expenses above provided for shall be held by the secretary as a special fund for meeting the expenses of said board ; he giving such bond as said board shall from time to time direct.

SEC. 4408. The Ohio board of pharmacy shall examine every person who desires to carry on or engage in the business of a retail apothecary or of retailing any drugs, medicines, chemicals, poisons, or pharmaceutical preparations, or of compounding or dispensing the prescriptions of physicians, as proprietor and manager, touching his competency and qualifications for that purpose, and upon a majority of the board being satisfied of such competency and qualification, they shall furnish such person a certificate of his competency and qualification as pharmacist, which certificate shall entitle the person named therein to conduct and carry on the business aforesaid as proprietor and manager thereof, upon complying with the requirements of section forty-four hundred and seven, and such board shall also examine each person who desires to engage in such business as assistant pharmacist, touching his competency and qualification, and upon any such person passing a satisfactory examination, shall furnish a certificate setting forth that he is a qualified assistant in pharmacy, which certificate shall enable the person named therein to engage in said business as an assistant pharmacist, upon his complying with the provisions of section forty-four hundred and seven.

SEC. 4409. The provisions of section forty-four hundred and eight shall not apply to any person engaged in the retail drug and apothecary business, as proprietor or manager of the same, at the time of the passage of this act, or who, being at the age of eighteen years, has been continuously employed or engaged for three years immediately preceding the passage of this act as assistant in any retail drug store in the United States, in the compounding or dispensing of medicines on the prescriptions of physicians, who has complied with the provisions of section forty-four hundred and seven.

SEC. 4410. No person, not a qualified assistant, shall be allowed by the proprietor or manager of any retail drug or chemical store to compound or dispense the prescriptions of physicians, except as an aid under the supervision of a registered pharmacist or his qualified assistant.

SEC. 4411. A qualified assistant, within the meaning of this chapter, shall be a clerk or assistant in a retail drug or chemical store who shall furnish to the Ohio board of pharmacy such evidence of his employment as is required by section forty-four hundred and seven, or a person holding the certificate of said board, as an assistant pharmacist, as provided in section forty-four hundred and eight; but it shall be unlawful for such assistant pharmacist, or qualified assistant, to supervise or manage any pharmacy or retail drug or chemical store, or to engage in the occupation of compounding or dispensing medicines on prescriptions of physicians, or selling at retail for medicinal purposes any drugs, chemicals, poisons, or pharmaceutical preparation except when engaged or employed in a pharmacy, retail drug or chemical store which is in charge of and is under the supervision and management of a registered pharmacist.

SEC. 4412. Any person owning a pharmacy, retail drug or chemical store, who, in violation of the provisions of section 4405 of this act, causes or permits the same to be conducted or managed by a person not a registered pharmacist, shall be deemed guilty of a misdemeanor, and upon conviction thereof shall be fined in any sum not less than twenty dollars nor more than one hundred dollars, and each week that he shall cause or permit such pharmacy, retail drug or chemical store to be so conducted or managed, shall constitute a separate and distinct offense and render him liable to separate prosecution and punishment therefor; a person violating the provisions of section forty-four hundred and seven, relating to registration, renewal of registration, or failing to conspicuously expose such certificate of registration shall be deemed guilty of a misdemeanor, and upon conviction thereof shall be fined in any sum not exceeding one hundred dollars for each week he continues to carry on or to be engaged in such business, without such registration or such exposure of such certificate of registration, or renewal thereof. And for the violation of any of the provisions of section forty-four hundred and ten, such proprietor or manager shall be deemed guilty of a misdemeanor, and upon conviction thereof shall be fined in any sum not exceeding fifty dollars for each and every offense; and for the violation of any of the provisions of forty-four hundred and eleven, such assistant pharmacist shall be deemed guilty of a misdemeanor, and upon conviction thereof shall be fined in any sum not exceeding fifty dollars for each and every offense. All fines assessed for the violation of any of the provisions of this act shall be placed in the county treasury for the use and benefit of the common-school fund of the county in which such offense is committed: *Provided,* That nothing in this act shall be so construed as to in any way affect the right of any person to bring a civil action against any person referred to in this act, for any act or acts for which a civil action may now be brought. It shall be the duty of the Ohio board of pharmacy, upon application therefor being made to said board, to cause the prosecution of any person or persons violating any of the provisions of this act.

## MORPHINE LAW.

SECTION 1. *Be it enacted by the General Assembly of the State of Ohio,* That it shall not be lawful for any person, other than a wholesale druggist or other dealer in drugs and medicines, to sell or offer for sale at wholesale, or for any person other than a registered pharmacist or a registered assistant pharmacist to sell or offer for sale at retail, morphine or any of its salts, in this State, and it shall not be lawful for such person to sell or offer for sale morphine or any of its salts in any bottle or vial, envelope, or other package, unless the same shall be wrapped in scarlet paper or envelope, and all bottles or vials used for the above purpose shall contain not more than one drachm each, and shall have, in addition to said scarlet wrapper, a scarlet label lettered in white letters, and the same must be upon both vial and wrapper, when vials are used, plainly naming the contents of said bottle; and further, that no person shall have the right to change any preparation of morphine from its original package to any other receptacle whatever for the purpose of retailing or dispensing therefrom, but it must be retailed or dispensed only from the original package with scarlet wrapper as aforesaid.

SEC. 2. That anyone violating the provisions of the above section shall be guilty of a misdemeanor, and on conviction thereof shall be fined not less than ten nor more than fifty dollars, at the discretion of the court, for each and every violation of the preceding section.

SEC. 3. That all laws and parts of laws in conflict with this act be, and the same are hereby repealed.

SEC. 4. This act shall take effect and be in force from and after September 1, 1886.

## LABEL LAW.

AN ACT to provide for the proper labeling of poisonous articles.

SECTION 1. *Be it enacted by the General Assembly of the State of Ohio,* That whenever any pharmacist, druggist, or other dealer in poisons, chemicals, medicines, and drugs, whether wholesale or retail, shall sell any drug or chemical an indiscriminate or careless use of which would be destructive of human life, such dealer shall affix to each bottle or package of such drug, chemical, or poison a label printed in red ink, having on it the name of the article by which it is commonly known, the cautionary emblem of the skull and crossbones, the words "caution" and "poison," and in addition thereto at least two of the most readily obtainable effective antidotes to such poisonous articles.

SEC. 2. Whoever violates the provisions of section one (1) of this act shall, upon conviction thereof before any court having competent jurisdiction, be fined in any sum not exceeding one hundred dollars nor less than ten dollars.

SEC. 3. This act shall take effect and be in force sixty days after its passage.

## POISON LAW.

Whoever sells or gives away any quantity of arsenic less than one pound without first mixing therewith soot or indigo in the proportion of one ounce of soot or half an ounce of indigo to the pound of arsenic, or except upon the prescription of a physician sells or gives away any quantity of any article belonging to the class usually denominated poisons, to any minor, or sells or gives away any such article to any person, without having first marked the word "poison" upon the label or wrapper containing the same and registered, in a book to be by him kept for that purpose, the day and date upon which it is sold or given away, the quantity thereof, the name, age, sex, and color of person obtaining the same, the purpose for which it is required, and the name and place of abode of the person for whom the same is intended, shall be fined not more than two hundred nor less than twenty dollars.

## PENNSYLVANIA.

AN ACT to regulate the practice of pharmacy and sale of poisons and to prevent adulterations in drugs and medicinal preparations in the State of Pennsylvania.

Whereas, the safety of the public is endangered by want of care in the sale of poisons, whether to be used as such for such legitimate purposes or employed as medicines and dispensed on the prescriptions of physicians;

And whereas, the ability of physicians to overcome disease depends greatly on their obtaining good and unadulterated drugs and properly prepared medicines;

And whereas, the persons to whom the preparation and sale of drugs, medicines, and poisons properly belong, known as apothecaries, chemists, and druggists or pharmacists, should possess a practical knowledge of the business and science of pharmacy in all its relations: Therefore,

SECTION 1. *Be it enacted by the Senate and House of Representatives of the Commonwealth of Pennsylvania in General Assembly met, and it is hereby enacted by the authority of the same,* That the first section of the act entitled "An act to regulate the practice of pharmacy and sale of poisons and to prevent adulterations in drugs and medicinal preparations in the State of Pennsylvania," approved the twenty-fourth day of May, anno domini one thousand eight hundred and eighty-seven, which reads as follows:

"SECTION 1. *Be it enacted by the Senate and House of Representatives of the Commonwealth of Pennsylvania in General Assembly met, and it is hereby enacted by the authority of the same,* That hereafter no person whomsoever shall open, or carry on as manager, in the State of Pennsylvania, any retail drug or chemical store, nor engage in the business of compounding or dispensing medicines or prescriptions of physicians, or of selling at retail any drugs, chemicals, poisons, or medicines, without having obtained a certificate of competency and qualification so to do from the State pharmaceutical examining board and having been duly registered as herein provided," shall be amended so as to read as follows:

SECTION 1. *Be it enacted by the Senate and House of Representatives of the Commonwealth of Pennsylvania in General Assembly met, and it is hereby enacted by the authority of the same,* That hereafter no person whomsoever shall open, or carry on as manager, in the State of Pennsylvania, any retail drug or chemical store, nor engage in the business of compounding or dispensing medicines or prescriptions of physicians, or of selling at retail any drugs, chemicals, poisons, or medicines, without having obtained a certificate of competency and qualification so to do from the State pharmaceutical examining board and having been duly registered as herein provided, but it shall be lawful for the widow or legal representatives of a deceased person who was a manager and registered pharmacist to carry on or continue the business of such deceased pharmacist: *Provided,* That the actual retailing, dispensing, or compounding of medicines or poisons be done only by an assistant qualified and registered as herein provided. *Any person who shall violate or fail to comply with the provisions of this section shall be guilty of a misdemeanor, and on conviction before any court shall be punished by a fine not exceeding one hundred dollars.*

Approved June 16th, 1891.

SEC. 2. That there shall be established in the State of Pennsylvania a board, to be styled the State pharmaceutical examining board, to consist of five persons, three of whom shall constitute a quorum, who shall be appointed by the governor from among the most skillful retail apothecaries actually engaged in said business in the State of Pennsylvania, and who must have had ten years' practical experience in the same—one to serve five years, one four years, one three years, one two years, and one one year in the first instance, and thereafter annually the governor shall appoint one person to serve as a member of said board for the term of five years. The said persons so appointed shall be and constitute the said the State pharmaceutical examining board, and shall hold the office for the term for which they were appointed, or until their successors are duly appointed and qualified, and shall receive as a compensation for their services five dollars for each day actually engaged in this service and all legitimate and necessary expenses incurred in attending the meetings of said board under the provisions of this act, and no part of the salary of said board or expenses thereof shall be paid out of the State treasury.

The said board shall organize by electing one of its members secretary, who in addition to his compensation as a member of said board shall receive a further sum, not to exceed one hundred dollars annually, for his services as secretary.

They, the said board, and each of them, shall, within ten days after their appointment or being apprised of the same, take and subscribe an oath or affirmation before a properly qualified officer of the county in which they reside that they will faithfully and impartially perform the duties of their office.

Any vacancies occurring in said board shall be filled by the governor of the State of Pennsylvania from among such only as are eligible for original appointment.

SEC. 3. The said pharmaceutical examining board shall keep a book of registration open at some convenient place, of which due notice shall be given by advertisement in at least four newspapers in the State, and so divided as to reach as nearly as practicable all parts thereof, in which book shall be registered the name and address of each and every person duly qualified under this act to conduct and carry on the retail drug and apothecary business or to hold the position of qualified assistant therein. And it shall be the duty of all persons now conducting, or who shall hereafter conduct, the business of retail apothecaries, or those acting in the capacity of qualified assistants therein in said State, to apply to said board and be registered as such within ninety days after such notice, and thereafter every three years. Application for registration only may be sent by mail to the secretary of the examining board after being properly attested before a notary public or any other person authorized to administer an oath or affirmation in the county in which the applicant resides.

The form of application shall be subject to such regulations as the board may see proper to adopt, but in no case shall the applicant be put to any unnecessary expense in order to secure registration.

SEC. 4. The said board shall be entitled to demand and receive from each applicant for examination and registration and for the certificate hereinafter provided a fee not to exceed two dollars, and for registration only a fee not to exceed one dollar in the first instance, and for renewing the same every three years a fee not to exceed one dollar; and the amount derived from this source shall be held by said board and be applied to the expenses and salaries herein provided and such as may arise under the provisions of this act, and they, the said board, shall report annually to the governor of the State of Pennsylvania all moneys received and disbursed under the provisions of this act, together with the number of pharmacists registered under this act.

SEC. 5. That it shall be the duty of said board to meet *at least* once every three months in the city of Harrisburg, or at such other place as they may deem expedient, and examine all persons who shall desire to carry on the business of a retail apothecary, or that of retailing drugs, chemicals, or poisons, or of compounding physicians' prescriptions, touching their competency and qualifications, and they, the said board, or a majority of them shall grant to such persons as may be qualified certificates of competency or qualification, which shall entitle the holders thereof either to conduct or carry on the business or to act as a qualified assistant therein, as may be expressed upon the said certificate, and such certificate, together with its renewals, shall be good and sufficient evidence of registration under this act.

All persons applying for examination for certificate to entitle them to conduct and carry on the retail drug or apothecary business must produce satisfactory evidence of having had not less than four years' practical experience in the business. And those applying for examination for certificates as qualified assistants therein must produce evidence of having not less than two years' experience in said business.

SEC. 6. That no person shall hereafter engage as manager in the business of an apothecary or pharmacist, or of retailing drugs, chemicals, and poisons, or of compounding and dispensing the prescriptions of physicians, either directly or indirectly, without having obtained such certificate as aforesaid. But nothing contained in this act shall in any manner whatever interfere with the business of any practitioner of medicine, nor prevent him from administering or supplying to his patients such articles as to him may seem fit and proper, nor shall it interfere with the making and dealing in proprietary remedies, popularly called patent medicines, nor prevent storekeepers from dealing in and selling the commonly used medicines and poisons, if such medicines and poisons conform in all respects to the requirements of section 9, provided the provisions of section 10 of this act be fully complied with.

Any person who shall violate or fail to comply with the provisions of this section shall be guilty of a misdemeanor, and on conviction before any court shall be punished by a fine not exceeding one hundred dollars, or be imprisoned in the county jail of the proper county for a term not exceeding one year, or either or both, at the discretion of the court.

SEC. 7. That the foregoing provisions of this act shall not apply to or affect any person who shall be engaged in the retail drug and apothecary business as proprietor of the same, or as qualified assistant therein at the passage of this act, except only in so far as relates to registration and fees provided in sections 3 and 4 of this act.

A qualified assistant, engaged in the business at the passage of this act, is one who has had not less than two years' practical experience in the retail drug and apothecary business. All other assistants actually engaged in the business at the passage of this act shall, upon the completion of a like term of two years' experience, be entitled to registration as qualified assistants without examination.

SEC. 8. That no person shall be allowed by the proprietor or manager of any store or place where prescriptions are compounded to compound or dispense the prescriptions of physicians except under the immediate supervision of said proprietor or his qualified assistant, unless holding a properly certified certificate of registration or competency from the state pharmaceutical examining board as herein provided, and any person violating the provisions of this section shall be deemed guilty of a misdemeanor, and on conviction thereof shall be punished by a fine not exceeding one hundred dollars.

SEC. 9. That no person shall knowingly, willfully, or fraudulently falsify or adulterate, or cause to be falsified or adulterated, any drug or medical substance or any preparation authorized or recognized by the pharmacopœia of the United States, or used or intended to be used in medicinal practice, nor mix or cause to be mixed with any such drug or medicinal substance any foreign or inert substance whatsoever, for the purpose of destroying or weakening its medicinal power and effect, and willfully, knowingly, or fraudulently sell or cause the same to be sold for medicinal purposes.

Any person who shall violate this section shall be deemed guilty of a misdemeanor, and upon conviction thereof shall be punished by a fine not exceeding five hundred dollars, and shall forfeit to the commonwealth all articles so adulterated.

SEC. 10. *Poisons.* — A poison in the meaning of this act shall be any drug, chemical, or preparation which, according to standard works on medicine or materia medica, is liable to be destructive to adult human life in quantities of sixty grains or less.

No person shall sell at retail any poisons except as herein provided, without affixing to the bottle, box, vessel, or package containing the same, a label, printed or plainly written, containing the name of the article, the word "poison," and the name and place of business of the seller; nor shall he deliver poison to any person without satisfying himself that such poison is to be used for legitimate purposes.

It shall be the further duty of anyone selling or dispensing poisons, which are known to be destructive to adult human life in quantities of five grains or less, before delivering them to enter in a book, kept for this purpose, the name of the seller, the name and residence of the buyer, the name of the article, quantity sold or disposed of, and the purpose for which it is said to be intended, which book of registry shall be preserved for at least two years, and shall at all times be open to the inspection of the coroner or courts of the county in which the same may be kept.

The provisions of this section shall not apply to the dispensing of physicians' prescriptions specifying poisonous articles, nor to the sale to agriculturists of such articles as are commonly used by them as insecticides. Any person failing to comply with the provisions of this section shall be deemed guilty of a misdemeanor, and upon conviction thereof shall be punished by a fine of not less than five nor more than fifty dollars for each and every offense.

\* SEC. 11. Repealed.

SEC. 12. It shall be the duty of the State pharmaceutical examining board to investigate all complaints and charges of noncompliance or violation of the provisions of this act, and prosecute all persons so offending whenever there shall appear to the board reasonable ground for such action.

SEC. 13. That all acts and parts of acts, so far as they may be in conflict with this, are hereby declared void and of no effect.

Approved May 24, 1887.

---

\*AN ACT to repeal Sec. 11 of an act entitled "An act to regulate the practice of pharmacy and sale of poisons, and to prevent adulterations in drugs and medicinal preparations in the State of Pennsylvania," approved the twenty-fourth day of May, anno Domini one thousand eight hundred and eighty-seven.

SECTION 1. *Be it enacted by the Senate and House of Representatives of the Commonwealth of Pennsylvania in General Assembly met,* and it is hereby enacted by the authority of the same, that section 11 of an act entitled "An act to regulate the practice of pharmacy and sale of poisons, and to prevent adulterations in drugs

# RHODE ISLAND.

### Chapter 131.—Of Medicines and Poisons.

Section 1. No person, unless a registered pharmacist or registered assistant pharmacist in the employ of a registered pharmacist, or unless acting as an aid under the immediate supervision of a registered pharmacist or a registered assistant pharmacist, within the meaning of this chapter, shall retail, compound, or dispense medicines or poisons, except as hereinafter provided.

Sec. 2. Every person in order to be a registered pharmacist or a registered assistant pharmacist, within the meaning of this chapter, shall be either a graduate in pharmacy, a practising pharmacist or a practising assistant in pharmacy. Graduates in pharmacy shall be such as have obtained a diploma from a regularly incorporated college of pharmacy and shall have presented satisfactory evidence of their qualifications to the State board of pharmacy. A practicing pharmacist shall be deemed to be a person, who, on the twenty-fourth day of March, one thousand eight hundred seventy-one, kept and continued thereafter to keep an open shop for compounding and dispensing the prescriptions of medical practitioners and for the retailing of drugs and medicines, and who shall give to the State board of pharmacy satisfactory evidence of his qualifications, and shall have declared his intention in writing of keeping open shop for the compounding of prescriptions and the retailing of drugs and medicines, and such other persons as shall have given to the State board of pharmacy satisfactory evidence of their qualifications, and shall have declared their intention in writing of keeping open shop for the compounding of prescriptions and the retailing of drugs and medicines. A practicing assistant in pharmacy shall be deemed to be a person who shall have served three years' apprenticeship in a shop where the prescriptions of medical practitioners are compounded, and shall have passed a satisfactory examination before the State board of pharmacy.

Sec. 3. The State board of pharmacy shall consist of seven persons, to be appointed by the governor from the registered pharmacists of the State, and shall hold office for the term of three years and until their successors are appointed, and in case of vacancy at any time, arising from resignation, death, or removal from the State, the governor may fill such vacancy from the registered pharmacists of the State. Four members of said board shall constitute a quorum. Said board shall organize by the election of a president and secretary, both of whom shall sign all certificates and other official documents. Said board shall meet twice a year, and may make by-laws and all necessary regulations, not repugnant to law, for the proper fulfilment of their duties. The presiding officer of said board may administer oaths in relation to all matters connected with or in the administration of the duties of the board. The secretary of said board shall also be registrar of pharmacists. The said board shall examine all applicants for registration, shall direct the registration by the registrar of all persons properly qualified or entitled thereto, and shall report annually to the general assembly on the condition of pharmacy, together with the names of all registered pharmacists and assistant pharmacists. The registrar of pharmacists shall keep a

---

and medicinal preparations in the State of Pennsylvania," approved the twenty-fourth day of May, anno Domini one thousand eight hundred and eighty-seven, which reads as follows: "Any graduate of an accredited medical college, who has had not less than three years' continuous practice since the date of his diploma, and who is registered as a practitioner of medicine and surgery under the act entitled 'An act to provide for the registration of all practitioners of medicine and surgery,' approved the eighth day of June, anno Domini one thousand eight hundred and eighty-one, may be registered under this act without examination, and be granted a certificate which shall entitle him to conduct and carry on the retail drug or apothecary business as proprietor or manager thereof, subject to fees provided in sections 3 and 4 of this act," be, and the same is hereby, repealed.

book in which shall be entered, under the supervision of the State board of pharmacy, the name and place of business of every person who shall apply for registration. The registrar shall note the fact against the name of any registered pharmacist or assistant pharmacist who may have died or removed from the State or disposed of or relinquished his business, and shall make all necessary alterations in the location of persons registered under this chapter.

SEC. 4. The certificate of the secretary of the State board of pharmacy and registrar of pharmacists as to any matter of record of said board or of the nonexistence of any matter in the record of said board, as to which said secretary may be called upon to testify in his official capacity, shall be admissible evidence in any court in this State of the existence or nonexistence of such matter. Said secretary shall be paid the sum of twenty-five cents for every such certificate, which sum shall be taxed in the costs of any proceedings pending in any court in which the same shall be offered as evidence.

SEC. 5. Every person applying for examination and registration shall pay to the State board of pharmacy ten dollars, and on passing the examination required shall be furnished, free of expense, with a certificate of registration. Every registered assistant pharmacist may, with the consent of said board, be entitled to registration as a registered pharmacist and shall be furnished with a certificate of registration, for which certificate he shall pay the registrar one dollar. Every certificate issued by said board shall be renewed annually, for which renewal one dollar shall be paid to the registrar. The fees received for examinations, registration, and certificates shall be appropriated to defray the expenses of the State board of pharmacy. The registration of every person registered by the board shall expire on the first day of July next ensuing the granting thereof; and if any person so registered shall not apply for a renewal of his registration on or before the first day of July, annually, the registrar of pharmacists shall note the fact against the name of such person, who shall thereafter cease to be a registered pharmacist or registered assistant pharmacist. Said board may, in their discretion, refuse to renew any such registration, and may at any time, for good and sufficient cause, discontinue any registration previously granted.

SEC. 6. The certificate issued by said board shall be used by the person to whom issued in but one place of business; but said board may permit such person in removing to another place of business to continue the use of such certificate with the same force and effect as in the place for which such certificate was issued. Such person removing shall notify said board of the change of his place of business, and failing so to do shall cease to be a registered pharmacist. No registered pharmacist shall be the proprietor of more than one place of business unless he shall at each place of business of which he is the proprietor, at all times when open, keep one or more registered pharmacists.

SEC. 7. Every person, not a registered pharmacist, who shall keep open shop for the retailing and dispensing of medicines and poisons, or who shall take, use, or exhibit the title of registered pharmacist, and every person who shall violate any of the provisions of this chapter shall, upon the first conviction, be fined fifty dollars and, upon the second and every subsequent conviction, shall be fined one hundred dollars; and all fines recovered shall enure, one-half thereof to the use of the State and one-half thereof to the use of the complainant: *Provided, however,* That in towns or parts of towns where there is no registered pharmacist within three miles, any person may sell the usual domestic medicines put up by a registered pharmacist, and marked with his label, such person procuring annually a certificate from the State board of pharmacy therefor, and paying one dollar for such certificate.

SEC. 8. Nothing hereinbefore contained shall apply to any practitioner of medicine who does not keep open shop for the retailing, dispensing, or compounding of medicines or poisons, nor prevent him from administering or supplying to his patients such articles as he may deem fit and proper; nor shall it interfere with the making and dealing in proprietary medicines, popularly called patent medicines, unless such medicines be wholly or in part composed of some of the articles enumerated in schedule A of this chapter, nor with the business of wholesale dealers in supplying medicines and poisons to registered pharmacists and physicians, and for use in the arts; nor shall it apply to such wholesale dealers in drugs and medicines in the trade on the twenty-sixth day of March, one thousand eight hundred and seventy-four, as the State board of pharmacy shall in their discretion deem suitable persons, and who shall keep and maintain in their employ one or more registered assistant pharmacists, who shall have the sole charge and care of the compounding and dispensing of all medicines and poisons sold at retail.

SEC. 9. No person shall hereafter sell, either by wholesale or retail, any of the poisons enumerated in schedule A of this chapter, without distinctly labeling the bottle, box, vessel, or paper and wrapper or cover in which said poison is contained, with the name of the article, the word poison, and the name and place of business of the seller; and every registered pharmacist selling or dispensing any of said poisons shall first enter in a book, to be kept for that purpose only, and subject always to inspection by the State board of pharmacy or any officer or agent thereof or other proper authority, and to be preserved for at least five years, a record of the same in accordance with schedule B of this chapter: *Provided*, That if any of said poisons form a part of the ingredients of any medicine or medicines compounded in accordance with the written prescription of a medical practitioner, the same need not be labeled with the word poison; but all prescriptions, whether or not composed in part or in whole of any of said ingredients, shall be carefully kept by the pharmacist on a file or in a book used for that purpose only and numbered in the order in which they are received or dispensed, and every box, bottle, vial, vessel, or packet containing medicines so dispensed shall be labeled with the name and place of business of the registered pharmacist so dispensing said medicine, and be numbered with a number corresponding with that on the original prescription retained by said pharmacist on such book or file. Such prescriptions shall be preserved at least five years, and shall be open to the inspection of the writer thereof, and a copy shall be furnished free of expense whenever demanded by either the writer or the purchaser thereof.

SEC. 10. Every person who shall knowingly adulterate or cause to be mixed any foreign or inert substance with any drug or medicinal substance, or any compound medicinal preparation recognized by the pharmacopœia of the United States or of other countries, as employed in medicinal practice, with the effect of weakening or destroying its medicinal power, or who shall sell the same knowing it to be adulterated, shall, in addition to the penalties prescribed in section seven hereof, forfeit to the use of the State all articles so adulterated found in his possession and shall be deprived of the right of practicing as a pharmacist in this State thereafter. Whenever complaint shall be made of any violation of the provisions of this section, the State board of pharmacy, on being notified thereof, shall make investigation of the same, employing competent persons when necessary to make analysis of the articles alleged to be adulterated; and if such complaint shall be substantiated said board shall assist in making prosecution against the respondent.

SCHEDULE A.

Arsenic and its preparations.
Cotton root and its preparations.
Corrosive sublimate.
Cyanide of potassium.
Ergot and its preparations.
Hydrocyanic acid.
Opium and its preparations, paregoric excepted.

Oxalic acid.
Savin.
Strychnia.
Volatile oil of bitter almonds, of pennyroyal, of savin, and of tansy.
Proprietary or secret medicines recommended, sold, or advertised as emmenagogues and parturients.

SCHEDULE B.

*Form in which registered pharmacists and retail dealers in poison shall keep their poison-book.*

| Date. | Name of purchaser. | Name and quantity of poison sold. | For what purpose said to be required. | Remarks. |
|---|---|---|---|---|
|  |  |  |  |  |

## SOUTH CAROLINA.

AN ACT of incorporation to incorporate the pharmaceutical association of the State of South Carolina.

SECTION 1. *Be it enacted by the Senate and House of Representatives of the State of South Carolina, now met and sitting in General Assembly, and by the authority of the same,* That G. J. Luhn, G. W. Aimar, C. F. Panknin, A. W. Eckel, B. F. Moise, E. S. Burnham, A. H. Schwacke, C. O. Michaelis, A. O. Barbot, E. H. Heinitsh, A. H. Davega, W. C. Fisher, A. E. Norman, W. C. McMillan, H. E. Heintsh, W. A. Gibson, W. H. Harbers, H. Baer, and their associates and successors, are hereby made and created a body politic and corporate, under the name and style of "The Pharmaceutical Association of the State of South Carolina."

SEC. 2. That the said corporation hereby created and established shall have succession of officers and members according to its by-laws, and shall have power to make by-laws not repugnant to the laws of the land, and to have, use, and keep a common seal, and the same to alter at will; to sue and be sued in any court in the State, and to have and enjoy every right, power, and privilege incident to such corporation; and it is hereby empowered to take, hold, retain, possess, and enjoy all such property, real and personal, as may be given, bequeathed, or devised to it, or may be acquired by the said corporation, by purchase, or in any other manner whatever: *Provided,* The amount so held shall not exceed the sum of twenty-five thousand dollars, and to sell, alien, transfer the same or any part thereof.

SEC. 3. That the association hereby incorporated shall elect annually four members, who, with two other persons to be appointed by the Medical College of the State of South Carolina, shall constitute a board of pharmaceutical examiners for the city of Charleston, to hold office for the term of one year. And the said association shall elect annually four members, who, with two other persons to be appointed by the medical faculty of the University of South Carolina, shall constitute a board of pharmaceutical examiners of the city of Columbia, to hold office for the term of one year. Any vacancy or vacancies occurring in the course of the year in either or both of the above-mentioned boards shall be temporarily filled by the appointment of the president of the said association. The said board shall be styled "The boards of pharmaceutical examiners," and shall meet respectively in Charleston and Columbia once every three months, and keep in session until the applicants who have previously made application to the secretary of the said association shall have been examined; and four members of either the said boards shall constitute a quorum for the transaction of business and the granting of licenses.

SEC. 4. That from and after the passage of this act the said board of pharmaceutical examiners shall alone possess and exercise all the powers heretofore given, and now possessed by the faculty of the Medical College of the State of South Carolina and the medical faculty of the University of South Carolina in respect to the license of pharmaceutists, apothecaries, and druggists.

SEC. 5. That every pharmaceutist, apothecary, or retail druggist who carries on and conducts the business of such occupation in this State after the expiration of three months from the passage of this act must have a license therefor from one of the above-named boards. And any person who shall, thereafter, carry on and conduct the business of said occupations, or any of them, without such license, shall be liable to indictment as for a misdemeanor, and, on conviction, subject to a fine not exceeding five hundred dollars, or imprisonment not exceeding six months.

SEC. 6. That before granting said license, except in cases hereinafter excepted, each applicant therefor shall undergo an examination, by and before that board to which the application is made, and of such nature as they shall require; but such examination must include the reading of manuscript prescriptions and explanation thereof, the discovery or detection of unusual doses of drugs, and especially poisons, the recognition and distinguishing of the various roots, barks, leaves, fruits, resins, and gums in common use, and the proper antidotes and mode of administration thereof for the different poisons.

SEC. 7. That no examination shall be required in case the applicant is a regular graduate in medicine or pharmacy of a school that is in the *"ad eundem"* of the University of South Carolina or the Medical College of the State of South Carolina; but such an applicant shall be entitled to a license upon furnishing evidence of his graduation satisfactory to either of the said boards, and upon payment of a fee of five dollars for the license. That in case the applicant undergoes examination, the charge for the same and granting the licenses shall not exceed ten dollars; one-half of which shall go, in case the applicant was examined before the Charleston board, to the Medical College of the State of South Carolina, and in case the applicant was examined in the city of Columbia, to the University of South Carolina; and the balance in both cases to the pharmaceutical association of the State of South Carolina.

SEC. 8. That it shall be the sole duty of the Pharmaceutical Association of the State of South Carolina to establish, carry on, and preserve in a book to be kept for the purpose a register of all pharmaceutists, apothecaries, and retail druggists in the State, including the names of persons registered, place of business, the fact whether the person registered be a graduate in medicine or pharmacy, or whether under license granted on examination, and any other matter of information the said association may see fit to add.

SEC. 9. That it shall be the duty of all licensed pharmaceutists, apothecaries, and retail druggists, by whichsoever of the said boards licensed, to have their names registered in manner aforesaid by the pharmaceutical association of the State of South Carolina, and to report annually, on or before the first day of November, of each year, to the said pharmaceutical association of the State of South Carolina, whether any, and if yea, what change has occurred within the then preceding year as to their respective places of business; and for omission or neglect of the requirements of this section, or any of them, they shall, respectively, incur a fine of twenty-five dollars; and for each and every registration or change thereof, the party so registered shall pay to the secretary of said association the sum of one dollar, which shall be their compensation for the services performed, in accordance with the provisions of this act.

SEC. 10. That it shall be the duty of the pharmaceutical association of the State of South Carolina to make a correct report to the general assembly of work done by them, in accordance with the provisions of this act, on or before the first day in December in each year.

SEC. 11. That every pharmaceutist, or other person selling any poison, shall be satisfied that the purchase is made for legitimate purposes, and shall keep a book in which shall be recorded every sale of the following articles, viz: Arsenic and its preparations, all metallic cyanides, and cyanides of potassium, tartar emetic, corrosive sublimate, aconite and its preparations, strychnine, and all other poisonous alkaloids and their salts, cantharides, ergot, hydrocyanic acid; the said record also to exhibit the name of the person to whom sold, place of his residence, and purpose of purchase as stated, which book shall be kept at all times subject to the inspection of the coroner of the county and the solicitor of the said association, or such other persons as either of them may designate.

SEC. 12. That all persons in this State engaged in business as pharmaceutists, apothecaries, or druggists, either in the wholesale or retail of drugs, shall, to every bottle, vial, box, or other package containing any poison named in the preceding section, or any one or more of the following articles, viz, oxalic acid, chloroform belladonna and its preparations, opium and all its preparations, except paregoric, digitalis and its preparations, henbane and its preparations, hemlock or conium, or any other article that may be added to this list by the pharmaceutical association of the State of South Carolina, securely attach a label, whereon shall be either printed or legibly written with red ink the name of the poison and the name of at least one antidote, with brief directions as to the mode of using the same: *Provided*, That nothing herein contained shall be construed to apply to the filling of prescriptions made by regular physicians: *And provided, further,* That it shall be the duty of the boards of pharmaceutical examiners or either of the said boards, on application at the time of registration, to furnish to the party registering a form of label for poisons.

SEC. 13. That this act shall not be construed to prevent merchants and shopkeepers from vending or exposing for sale medicines already prepared: *Provided*, Such merchants and shopkeepers shall attach to the article sold a copy of the label attached thereto by wholesale druggists, and in the sale of poisons shall comply with the provisions of sections 11 and 12 of this act.

SEC. 14. That it shall not be lawful for the proprietor of any pharmaceutical shop to allow any person not qualified in accordance with the provisions of this act to dispense of poisons or compound the prescriptions of physicians; and any person who, upon an indictment for a violation of this section, shall be convicted of the same, shall pay a fine not exceeding five hundred dollars, or suffer imprisonment for a period of not more than six months.

SEC. 15. That this act shall not be construed so as in any way whatsoever, to affect those who have, previous to the date of the passage of the same, obtained a license from the medical faculty of the University of South Carolina, or the faculty of the Medical College of the State of South Carolina, nor in any way deprive the said faculties of granting diplomas to pharmaceutists, apothecaries, and druggists, who may have duly graduated in the Medical College of the State of South Carolina, or the medical department of the University of South Carolina, respectively, by virtue of which the said graduates shall be entitled to license without examination, upon payment of a fee of five dollars as above mentioned.

SEC. 16. That the said association is hereby authorized through and by its solicitor, or otherwise, as it may deem most expedient, to prosecute all persons violating the provisions of this act, or any of them.

SEC. 17. That all acts or parts of acts inconsistent with or repugnant to this act are hereby repealed.

Approved, March 10, 1876.

The following amendment to the act of incorporation was passed, to go into effect 1st May, A. D. 1882.

### SECTION 935, GENERAL STATUTES.

The said association is hereby authorized and directed to prosecute all persons violating the provisions of this chapter or any of them.

In case any person convicted of violating any of the provisions of this chapter, be punished by fine, one-half of said fine shall be paid to the informer, through whose agency such conviction shall be had.

# SOUTH DAKOTA.

CHAPTER 132.—[H. B. 104.]—CREATING A SOUTH DAKOTA PHARMACEUTICAL ASSOCIATION.

AN ACT creating a South Dakota pharmaceutical association; establishing a State board of pharmacy, and regulating the practice of pharmacy in the State.

*Be it enacted by the Legislature of the State of South Dakota:*

SECTION 1. *Name of association — board of pharmaceutical examiners — how appointed.*—The registered pharmacists in this State are hereby constituted an association under the name and title of the South Dakota pharmaceutical association, the purpose of which shall be to improve the science and art of pharmacy, and to restrict the sale of medicines to regularly educated and qualified persons, as provided in this act. Said association shall hold its first annual meeting under the provisions of this act at Yankton on the first Wednesday in August, 1893, and annually thereafter at such time and place as may be determined by the said association. The South Dakota pharmaceutical association shall report annually to the governor, recommending the names of at least three (3) members from the district in which the annual vacancy occurs, as persons qualified to be appointed upon said board, and the persons so appointed shall constitute the State board of pharmaceutical examiners for South Dakota, and shall hold their office for the term of three (3) years, or until their successors are appointed and qualified: *Provided,* That each member of said board shall be a practicing pharmacist, doing a retail drug business in this State: *And provided further,* That the appointments on said board shall be made by the governor on or before the first day of October in each year from among the members recommended by said association, one person from each pharmaceutical district as now existing, and the term of office for each member of said board shall be for three years: *Provided further,* That the State board of pharmaceutical examiners as now constituted shall continue until their successors in office are appointed and qualified as provided further in this act. All other vacancies shall be filled by the governor from the nominees last submitted residing in the district where such vacancy occurs: *Provided further,* That the State may be redistricted at any future annual meeting of the association, notice of the contemplated change having been sent to the members of the association by the secretary of the board at the same time notice of the annual meeting is mailed.

SEC. 2. *Secretary and treasurer—bond of—duties.*—The secretary and treasurer of the South Dakota pharmaceutical association shall each respectively be secretary and treasurer of the board of pharmacy and they shall each give such bonds as the association may require. The secretary shall pay over to the treasurer all moneys that shall come into his hands as such secretary, and the treasurer shall disburse the same only on order of the president of the association countersigned by the secretary. It shall be the duty of the board to examine all applications for registration submitted in due form, as provided in the rules and regulations of the board, to grant certificates of registration to such persons as may be entitled to the same under the provisions of this act, and each member of the board shall investigate all charges brought to his notice in his district, and if in his judgment the charges can be sustained, shall make complaint to the proper prosecuting officer.

SEC. 3. *Meetings of board—reports—examination and registration of applicants.*— The board shall hold meetings for the examination of applicants for registration and the transaction of such other business as shall pertain to its duties, at such times and places as the South Dakota pharmaceutical association may direct: *Provided,* That special meetings of the board may be held whenever it shall be deemed necessary by a majority of the members thereof. It shall be the duty of the board to report annually to the governor and to the South Dakota pharmaceutical association upon the condition of pharmacy in this State, which said report shall also furnish a record of the proceedings of the said board for the year and also the names of all the pharmacists duly registered under this act. Said board shall have power to make by-laws and regulations for the proper fulfillment of its duties under this act and shall keep a book of registration in which shall be entered the names and places of business of all persons registered under this act, which book shall also, specify such facts as such persons shall claim to justify their registration. Two (2) members of said board shall constitute a quorum.

SEC. 4. *Who entitled to be registered pharmacists.*—Any person of good moral character and temperate habits, shall, upon approval of this board, be entitled to be registered as a pharmacist within the meaning of this act, who shall be a licentiate in pharmacy or who shall be a graduate from a reputable college of pharmacy, whose course of study and requirements are approved by the board of pharmaceutical examiners hereinafter provided for: *Provided,* That nothing in this act shall be construed to invalidate any certificate of registration now in force in this State.

SEC. 5. *Qualifications—certificate of registration.*—Licentiates in pharmacy shall be such persons, not less than eighteen years of age, who have had three years' experience in the practice of pharmacy or who shall hold a diploma from such medical college as shall be approved by the board, and have passed a satisfactory examination before the State board of pharmacy herein mentioned. The said board may in their discretion, grant certificates of registration to such persons as shall furnish with their application satisfactory proof that they have been registered by examination in some other State: *Provided,* That such other State shall require a degree of competency equal to that required of applicants in this State, and said board may also in their discretion under such rules and regulations as may be made by them, issue to applicants for an examination temporary certificates which shall be valid only until the next regular meeting of the board.

SEC. 6. *Assistant pharmacist—qualifications of.*—Any person shall be entitled to registration as assistant pharmacist who is of the age of eighteen years, of good moral character, temperate habits and has had two years of experience in the practice of pharmacy under a registered pharmacist, and shall pass an examination before the State board of pharmacy that shall show competency or qualification equal to such experience, or who shall hold a certificate of registration as such assistant from the South Dakota board of pharmacy, at the time this act takes effect. Any registered assistant pharmacist shall have the right to compound medicines or sell poisons under the direct supervision of a registered pharmacist, and he may take charge of a drug store or pharmacy during the temporary absence of the owner or manager thereof: *Provided,* That nothing herein shall be construed as giving such assistant authority to continuously perform any of the duties herein mentioned, except under the supervision and in the presence of the manager.

SEC. 7. *Registration fee.*—Every person applying for registration as a registered pharmacist or registered assistant pharmacist, shall pay with his application five ($5.00) dollars, and if upon examination certificate be not granted, the secretary shall refund to the applicant three ($3.00) dollars.

SEC. 8. *Renewal of certificate.*—Every registered pharmacist or registered assistant pharmacist shall annually thereafter on such date as the South Dakota pharmaceutical association may determine, pay to the secretary an annual registry fee to be fixed by the said association, which in no case shall exceed the sum of five dollars, for which he shall receive from the board of pharmacy a renewal of his certificate of registration. The failure of any registered pharmacist or registered assistant pharmacist to pay said fee within one year from the date of the expiration of his certificate, shall deprive him of the right of such renewal. Every certificate of registration or the renewal thereof granted under this act shall by the person to whom granted be posted in a conspicuous place in the pharmacy to which it applies.

SEC. 9. *Salary of secretary.*—The secretary of the association shall receive a salary which shall be fixed by the association. He shall also receive his traveling and other necessary expenses incurred in the performance of his official duties. The members of the board shall receive the sum of five ($5.00) dollars for each day actually engaged in its service and all legitimate and necessary expenses incurred in attending the meetings of said board. Said expenses shall be paid from the fees and penalties received by the association under the provision of this act.

SEC. 10. *Adulteration of drugs unlawful.*—No person shall add to or remove from any drug, medicines, chemical, or pharmaceutical preparation any ingredient or material for the purpose of adulteration or substitution, which will alter the nature or composition of such drugs or other preparation. Any person who shall thus wilfully adulterate or alter, or shall sell or offer for sale any such adulterated or altered preparation or cause to be substituted one material for another with the intention to defraud or deceive the purchaser, shall be deemed guilty of a misdemeanor and be liable to prosecution under this act.

SEC. 11. *Who may conduct pharmacy; penalty for violation.*—That it shall hereafter be unlawful for any person other than a registered pharmacist to retail, compound, or dispense drugs, medicines, or poisons or to open or conduct any pharmacy or store for retailing, compounding, or dispensing drugs, medicines, or poisons unless such person shall be a registered pharmacist within the meaning of this act, except as herein provided; and any person not being a registered pharmacist within the meaning of this act, who shall keep a pharmacy or store for retailing or compounding medicines or who shall take, use, or exhibit the title of a registered pharmacist, shall be deemed guilty of a misdemeanor and for each and every offense shall be punished by a fine of fifty ($50) dollars upon conviction thereof. Any registered pharmacist who shall permit the compounding or dispensing of prescriptions or the vending of drugs or poisons in his store or place of business except under the supervision of a registered pharmacist, or except by a registered assistant pharmacist as herein provided, or any pharmacist or assistant who, while continuing in business, shall fail or neglect to procure his annual registration, or any person who shall wilfully make any false representations to procure registration for himself or any other person, shall be deemed guilty of a misdemeanor and punished by a fine of not less than fifty ($50.00) dollars upon conviction thereof: *Provided,* That nothing in this act shall apply to or in any manner interfere with the business of any physician or prevent him from supplying to his patients such articles as may seem to him proper, and, *Provided, further,* That no part of this section shall be so construed as to give the right to any physician to furnish any intoxicating liquors to be used as a beverage on prescription or otherwise.

SEC. 12. *Shall keep register of poisons sold and to whom.*—No person shall sell any poison named in schedule "A" by retail unless the box, bottle, wrapper, or cover in which the poison is contained is distinctly labeled with the name of the article, the name and address of the person selling and the word poison, and no person shall sell any poison named in schedule "B" to any person unknown to the seller, unless introduced by some person known to the seller, and on every sale the seller shall, before delivery, make entry in a book kept for that purpose, stating the date of sale, the name and address of the purchaser, the name and quantity of the article sold, the purpose for which it is required, and the name of the person, if any, who introduced them. Any person failing to comply with the requirements of this section shall be deemed guilty of a misdemeanor and upon conviction thereof shall be fined ten ($10.00) dollars for every such omission.

SEC. 13. *Penalty for neglect of duty.*—Any member of the board of pharmacy or officer therein provided for, who shall willfully neglect any of the duties provided for in this act, or who shall aid or abet any person in the evasion or violation of this act, shall be deemed guilty of a misdemeanor, and upon conviction thereof shall be fined not less than fifty ($50.00) dollars for each and every offense, and any person violating any provision of this act shall be guilty of a misdemeanor and fined not less than fifty ($50.00) dollars, unless otherwise provided in this act.

SEC. 14. *Board may revoke certificate—when.*—Whenever the board of pharmacy shall be satisfied that any person holding a certificate of registration is for any reason incompetent or disqualified to perform the duties of a registered pharmacist as contemplated by the provisions of this act they shall have power to revoke their certificate: *Provided, however,* That such certificate shall not be cancelled except after a hearing before said board, at which a majority of its members shall be present and of which meeting the person holding the certificate to be cancelled shall have not less than ten days' notice, and then only upon due proof by examination or otherwise:. *Provided, further,* That an appeal from the decision of said board may be taken to the circuit court of the county in which the person whose certificate is cancelled resides in the same manner as is now provided by law in cases of appeal from the decision of county commissioners.

SEC. 15. *Penalties inure to whom.*—All penalties collected under the provisions of this act shall inure to the South Dakota pharmaceutical association.

SEC. 16. *Repeal.*—All acts and parts of acts in conflict with this act are hereby repealed.

SEC. 17. *Emergency.*—That an emergency is hereby declared to exist and, therefore, this act shall take effect and be in force from and after its passage and approval.

### SCHEDULE "A."

Acetate of lead, Paris green, oxalic acid, carbolic acid, chloral hydrate, chloroform, ether, sulphate of zinc, and other poisonous medicines fatal to human life in doses of from fifteen to sixty grains.

### SCHEDULE "B."

Aconite, arsenic, belladonna, opium (except in paragoric and Dover's powders) and their preparations, strychnine, corrosive sublimate, prussic acid, cyanide of potassium, nitric and sulphuric acids, tartar emetic, and other poisonous medicines fatal to human life in doses of fifteen grains or less.

Approved March 1, 1893.

## TENNESSEE.

### THE PHARMACY ACT.

AN ACT to establish a State board of pharmacy, and to regulate the practice of pharmacy, the sale of poisons, and to prohibit the adulteration of drugs in the State of Tennessee.

SECTION 1. *Be it enacted by the General Assembly of the State of Tennessee,* That from and after the passage of this act it shall be unlawful for any person, not a registered pharmacist, within the meaning of this act, to open or conduct any pharmacy or retail drug or chemical store as proprietor thereof, unless he shall have in his employ and place in charge of such pharmacy or retail drug or chemical store a registered pharmacist within the meaning of this act, who shall have the supervision and management of that part of the business requiring pharmaceutical skill and knowledge, or to engage in the occupation of compounding or dispensing medicines or prescriptions of physicians, or of selling at retail for medical purposes any drugs, chemicals, poisons, or pharmaceutical preparations within this State until he has complied with the provisions of this act: *Provided,* That nothing in this section shall apply to or in any manner interfere with the business of any physician, or prevent him supplying to his patients such articles as may seem to him proper, or with the making of patent or proprietary medicines, or with the selling by any country store of copperas, camphor, borax, blue vitriol, saltpeter, sulphur, brimstone, licorice, sage, quinine, juniper berries, senna leaves, castor oil, spirits of turpentine, sweet oil, glycerin, Glauber's salt, Epsom salts, cream of tartar, bicarbonate of sodium, and of paregoric, essence of peppermint, essence of cinnamon, essence of ginger, hive syrup, syrup of ipecac, tincture of arnica, syrup of tolu, syrup of squills, spirits of camphor, number six, sweet spirits of niter, compound cathartic pills, and other similar preparations when compounded by a regular pharmacist and put up in bottles and boxes bearing the label of such pharmacist or wholesale druggist, with the name of the article and directions for its use on each bottle or box, or with the exclusively wholesale business of any dealer.

SEC. 2. The executive committee of the Tennessee State druggists' association shall, immediately upon the passage of this act, submit to the governor the names of ten persons, residents of this State, who have had at least ten years' experience as pharmacists and druggists, and from the names so submitted to him the governor may select and appoint five persons who shall constitute a board to be styled The Tennessee board of pharmacy; and any member of the board may be removed by the governor for good cause shown him. One member of said board shall be appointed and hold his office one year, one for two years, one for three years, one for four years, and one for five years, and until their successors shall be appointed and qualified; and at its regular annual meeting in each and every year thereafter the said Tennessee State druggists' association shall select and submit to the governor the names of five persons, with the qualification hereinbefore mentioned, and the governor shall select and appoint from the names so submitted, or other qualified persons, one member of said board, who shall hold his office for five years, and until his successor shall have been appointed and qualified. Any vacancy that may occur in said board shall be filled for the unexpired term by the governor upon the recommendation of the remaining members of the board. Each member of said board shall, within ten days after his appointment, take and subscribe an oath or affirmation before a competent officer to faithfully and impartially perform the duties of his office.

SEC. 3. The Tennessee board of pharmacy shall hold one regular meeting each year at Nashville, and such additional meetings at such times and places as may be determined upon by said board, at each of which meetings it shall transact such business as is required by law; said board shall make such rules, by-laws, and regulations as may be necessary for the proper discharge of its duties, and shall make a report of proceedings, including an itemized account of all moneys received and expended by said board, pursuant to this act, and a list of the names of all the pharmacists duly registered under this act to the secretary of state on or before the 15th day of November, ———, and annually thereafter, and to the Tennessee State druggists' association. Said board shall keep a book of registration open at some place in Nashville, of which due notice shall be given in three or more newspapers of general circulation in the State, in which the name and place of business of every person duly qualified under this act to conduct or engage in the business mentioned and described in section 1 shall be registered. Every person now conducting or engaged in such business in this State as proprietor or manager of the same, or who, being of the age of 21 years, has been employed or engaged for five years preceding the passage of this act as an assistant in any retail drug store in the United States in the compounding and dispensing of medicines on the prescriptions of physicians, who shall furnish satisfactory evidence in writing and under oath of such facts within three months after the publication of said notice, shall be registered as a pharmacist without examination. Every person who has attained the age of 18 years, and who has been continually engaged in the United States for three years prior to the passage of this act, who shall present satisfactory evidence of the same within three months after the publication of said notice, shall be registered as an assistant pharmacist without examination. Every person who shall desire hereafter to conduct or engage in such business in this State shall appear before said board and be registered within ten days after receiving a certificate of competency and qualification of said board. The said board shall demand and receive from each person registered as a pharmacist a fee of not exceeding $2, and for a certificate as assistant pharmacist a fee of not exceeding $1, to be applied to the payment of expenses arising under the provisions of this act. Every registered pharmacist or assistant pharmacist who desires to continue the practice of his profession shall annually thereafter during the time he shall continue in such practice, on such date as said board may determine, pay to the secretary of said board a registration fee, to be fixed by said board, but which shall in no case exceed, if a pharmacist, $1, if assistant pharmacist, 50 cents, for which he shall receive a renewal of said registration. Every certificate of registration granted under this act shall be conspicuously exposed in the drug or chemical store to which it applies, or in which the assistant is engaged. The secretary of said board shall receive a salary which shall be fixed by the board; he shall also receive his traveling and other expenses incurred in the performance of his official duties. The other members of said board shall receive the sum of $3 for each day actually engaged in the service thereof, and all legitimate and necessary expenses incurred in attending the meetings of said board. Said salary, per diem and expenses, shall be paid after an itemized statement of the same has been rendered and approved by the board, from the fees and penalties received by said board under the provisions of this act. All moneys received in excess of said per diem allowance and other expenses above provided for shall be held by the secretary as a special fund for meeting the expenses of said board, he giving such bond as said board may from time to time direct.

SEC. 4. The Tennessee board of pharmacy shall examine every person who shall desire to carry on or engage in the business of a retail apothecary or of retailing any drugs, medicines, chemicals, poisons, or pharmaceutical preparations, or of compounding or dispensing the prescriptions of physicians as proprietor or manager, touching his competency and qualifications for that purpose and upon a majority of the board being satisfied of such qualifications, and upon the payment by the applicant of an examination fee of $5, they shall furnish the person a certificate of his competency and qualification as a pharmacist, which certificate shall entitle the person therein named to carry on the business aforesaid as proprietor or manager thereof upon complying with the requirements of section 3; and such board shall also examine each person who desires to engage in such business as assistant pharmacist touching his competency and qualification, and upon such person passing a satisfactory examination, and upon the payment by the applicant of an examination fee of $3 they shall furnish him a certificate setting forth that he is a qualified assistant in pharmacy, which certificate shall enable the person therein named to engage in said business as an assistant pharmacist upon his complying with section 3.

SEC. 5. The provisions of section 4 shall not apply to any person engaged in the retail drug and apothecary business as proprietor or manager of the same at the time of the passage of this act, or who, being of the age of 18 years, has been continuously employed or engaged for three years immediately preceding the passage of this act as an assistant in any retail drug store in the United States in the compounding or dispensing of medicines on the prescriptions of physicians, who have complied with the provisions of section 3.

SEC. 6. No person not a qualified assistant shall be allowed by proprietor or manager of a retail drug or chemical store to compound or dispense the prescriptions of a physician except as an aid under the supervision of a registered pharmacist or his qualified assistant.

SEC. 7. A qualified assistant within the meaning of this act shall be a clerk or an assistant in a retail drug or chemical store, who shall furnish to the Tennessee board of pharmacy such evidence of his employment as required in section 3, or a person holding a certificate of said board as an assistant pharmacist, as provided by section 4, but it shall be unlawful for an assistant pharmacist or qualified assistant to supervise or manage any pharmacy or retail drug or chemical store, or to engage in the occupation of compounding or dispensing of medicines on the prescriptions of physicians, or for selling at retail for medicinal purposes any drugs, chemicals, poisons, or pharmaceutical preparations, except when engaged or employed in a pharmacy, retail drug or chemical store which is in charge of and under the supervision and management of a regular pharmacist.

SEC. 8. Any person owning a pharmacy, retail drug or chemical store, who, in violation of the provisions of section 1 of this act, causes or permits the same to be conducted by a person not a registered pharmacist shall be deemed guilty of a misdemeanor, and upon conviction thereof shall be fined in any sum not less than $20 nor more than $100, and that each week he shall cause or permit such pharmacy, retail drug or chemical store, to be so conducted or managed, shall constitute a separate and distinct offense and render him subject to a separate prosecution and punishment. Therefore, a person violating the provisions of section 3 relating to registration, or failing to conspicuously expose such certificate of registration, shall be deemed guilty of a misdemeanor, and upon conviction thereof shall be fined in any sum not exceeding $50 for each and every offense; and for the violation of any of section 7 such assistant pharmacist shall be deemed guilty of a misdemeanor, and upon conviction thereof shall be fined in any sum not exceeding $50 for each and every offense. All fines assessed for the violation of any of the provisions of this act shall be placed in the hands of the secretary of the board of pharmacy to meet the necessary and legitimate expenses of the Tennessee board of pharmacy: *Provided,* That nothing in this act shall be construed as to in any way affect the right of any person to bring a civil action against any person referred to in this act, or for any act or acts for which a civil action may now be brought. It shall be the duty of the Tennessee board of pharmacy, upon application being made to said board, to cause the prosecution of any person or persons violating any of the provisions of this act.

Sec. 9. It shall be unlawful for any pharmacist, assistant pharmacist, or proprietor of any retail drug or chemical store, to fraudulently adulterate any drug, chemical, or medicine he may sell or dispense, and should be* knowingly, intentionally, or fraudulently adulterate, or cause to be adulterated, such drugs, chemicals, or medical preparations, he shall be deemed guilty of a misdemeanor, and upon conviction thereof shall be liable to a penalty not to exceed $100, and in addition thereto his name shall be stricken from the register.

Sec. 10. This act shall not apply to physicians putting up their own prescriptions.

Sec. 11. The provisions of this act shall only apply to cities and towns having over 3,200 inhabitants, the population always to be computed by reference to the last Federal census.

Sec. 12. All acts and parts of acts in conflict with this act are hereby repealed.

Sec. 13. This act shall take effect from and after the date of its passage, the public welfare requiring it.

## TEXAS.

AN ACT to regulate the practice of pharmacy in the State of Texas and providing penalty for the enforcement of the same.

Section 1. *Be it enacted by the Legislature of the State of Texas,* That it shall be unlawful for any person, unless a qualified pharmacist within the meaning of this act, to open or conduct any pharmacy or store for compounding medicines, or for anyone not a qualified pharmacist to prepare physicians' prescriptions or compound medicines, except under the direct supervision of a qualified pharmacist, as hereinafter provided.

Sec. 2. Any person, in order to be qualified, shall be twenty-one years old and shall have passed a satisfactory examination before the board of pharmacy of Texas, or shall be a graduate in pharmacy or an assistant in pharmacy.

Sec. 3. Graduates in pharmacy shall be such as have obtained a diploma from a regular incorporated college of pharmacy, and that requires not less than two years' experience in stores where prescriptions of medical practitioners have been compounded, before said diploma is issued.

Sec. 4. Assistants in pharmacy must be twenty-one years old and have had two years' experience in stores where prescriptions of medical practitioners have been prepared, and shall have passed a satisfactory examination before the board of pharmacy of Texas.

---

*Intended, doubtless, for "he."

SEC. 5. As soon as convenient after this act the presiding judge of the district court of the several judicial districts shall as soon as practicable severally appoint a board of pharmaceutical examiners for their respective districts, who shall hold their office two years, which appointment shall be in writing and signed by the judge making the same, and delivered to the person appointed. Said board of pharmaceutical examiners shall be composed of not less than three qualified pharmacists who are residents of the districts of which they are appointed. If a vacancy occurs in said board another shall be appointed as aforesaid to fill the unexpired term. Said board shall have power to make by-laws and all the necessary regulations for the proper fulfillment of their duties under this act.

SEC. 6. The board shall meet within ninety days after the passage of this act, and once a year thereafter, in as central portions of the district as practicable, and shall give one month's notice, through the public press, of the time and place of such meeting. The board shall organize for business by electing a registrar of pharmacy. The duties of said board shall be to examine all applicants for registration, to direct the registration by the registrar of all persons properly qualified or entitled thereto.

SEC. 7. The duties of the registrar of pharmacy shall be to keep a book in which shall be entered, under the supervision of the board of pharmacy, the name and place of business of every person who shall apply for registration, and a statement, signed by the person making the application, of such facts in the case as may claim to justify his or her application. It shall also be the duty of the registrar to duly note the fact against the name of any qualified pharmacist who may have died or removed from the State, or disposed of or relinquished his business.

SEC. 8. Any person, in order to become a qualified pharmacist within the meaning of this act, shall apply and appear for examination and registration, and shall pay to the board of pharmacy five dollars; and on passing the examination required shall be furnished, free of cost, a certificate of registration, signed by the said board. Should said person fail to pass a satisfactory examination he may at any one other meeting of the board of pharmacy, within twelve months, be permitted to be examined without cost.

SEC. 9. Graduates, as specified in section 3, shall apply for registration, and if they produce satisfactory evidence to the board of pharmacy that they have a right to be registered, shall, upon paying the said board three dollars, be furnished a certificate of registration without examination.

SEC. 10. Proprietors who are actively engaged in the preparation of physicians' prescriptions and compounding and vending medicine in the State of Texas at the passage of this act shall be exempt from examination; also assistants who are likewise engaged and have been so engaged for three years, and are twenty-one years old, provided he, she, or they will register, as specified in this act, at first meeting of the board of pharmacy, and upon paying the board three dollars shall be furnished with a certificate of registration: *Provided*, That the provisions of this bill shall not prevent any person from engaging in the business herein described as proprietors or owners thereof, provided such proprietor or owner shall have employed in his business some qualified pharmacist to fill his prescriptions and compound drugs.

SEC. 11. All persons receiving a certificate of registration shall place it in a conspicuous place in their place of business. In failing to do this, the board of pharmarcy shall cancel their registration and deprive them of their certificate.

SEC. 12. Any person not a qualified pharmacist, but continues to compound prescriptions or retail medicine without complying with this act, shall, upon first conviction, be sentenced to pay a fine of not less than fifty nor more than one hundred dollars; and upon the second and every subsequent conviction shall be sentenced to a fine of not less than one hundred nor more than two hundred dollars.

SEC. 13. Any person who shall procure registration for himself or for another under this act by making or causing to be made any false representation shall be guilty of a misdemeanor and shall be fined not less than twenty-five nor more than one hundred dollars, and the name of the person so fraudulently registered shall be stricken from the register.

SEC. 14. Any member of the board of pharmacy may issue temporary certificates upon satisfactory proof that the applicant is competent; but said temporary certificate shall be null and void after the first regular or extra meeting of the board next after granting said temporary certificate: *Provided, further*, That not more than one temporary certificate shall ever be granted to any one person.

SEC. 15. All courts having jurisdiction in criminal causes are required to give this act in charge to each grand jury impannelled in such courts.

SEC. 16. This act shall not apply to towns and cities containing less than 1,000 inhabitants. Towns and cities that arrive at one or more thousand inhabitants on and after the passage of this act shall come within its provisions. The manner of ascertaining the census shall be the last official one, whether it be Federal, State, town, or city.

SEC. 17. Nothing in this act shall be construed to apply to any practitioner of medicine who does not keep open shop for compounding, dispensing, and selling medicine; nor so construed as to prevent any person or persons from investing their means in a drug store or stores, provided they keep employed qualified pharmacists for the direct supervision of vending and compounding medicines.

SEC. 18. The near approach of the close of the present session of the legislature and the great improbability of reaching this bill in its regular call, and the great importance for legislation on the subject embraced in this bill creates an emergency and a public necessity requiring the suspension of the constitutional rule requiring bills to be read on three several days before suspended, and it is so suspended, and that this act take effect and be in force from and after its passage, and it is so enacted.

## UTAH.

### AN ACT regulating the practice of pharmacy.

*Be it enacted by the Governor and Legislative Assembly of the Territory of Utah:*

SECTION 1. That it shall not be lawful for any person other than a registered pharmacist to compound or dispense drugs, medicines, or poisons, or to open or conduct any pharmacy for compounding or dispensing drugs, medicines, or poisons, unless such persons shall be or shall employ and place in charge of said pharmacy or store a registered pharmacist within the meaning of this act, except as hereinafter provided.

SEC. 2. Any person shall be entitled to be registered as a registered pharmacist within the meaning of this act who shall be a licentiate in pharmacy or shall furnish evidence to the Territorial board of pharmacy, hereinafter mentioned, that he has had four years' experience in compounding drugs in a store or pharmacy where the prescriptions of medical practitioners are compounded. The said board shall have the right to refuse registration to applicants whose examination or credentials are not satisfactory evidence of their competency. This provision shall also apply to the registration of assistant pharmacists hereinafter mentioned.

SEC. 3. Graduates in pharmacy who have obtained diplomas from such colleges or schools of pharmacy as shall be approved of by the board of pharmacy, and who, previous to obtaining said diplomas, have had three years' practical experience in a drug store where physicians' prescriptions are compounded and dispensed, may, on payment of a fee hereinafter provided, be made registered pharmacists.

SEC. 4. Licentiates in pharmacy shall be such persons as have had four years' practical experience in drug stores wherein prescriptions of medical practitioners are compounded and are not less than eighteen years of age, and have sustained a satisfactory examination before the Territorial board of pharmacy, and shall be granted a certificate accordingly upon the payment of a fee hereinafter named.

SEC. 5. It shall be the duty of said board of pharmacy to grant an assistant's certificate to such persons as have had two years' practical experience in drug stores where prescriptions of medical practitioners are compounded, and have passed a satisfactory examination before said board of pharmacy. The holder of said certificate shall have the right to act as clerk or salesman during the temporary absence of the owner or manager thereof.

SEC. 6. Immediately upon the passage of this act, the governor of the Territory of Utah shall, by and with the consent of the legislative council, appoint five (5) persons from among such competent pharmacists that have had five years' practical experience in the capacity of dispensing pharmacists, selecting not more than two members from any one city, and the said five pharmacists shall constitute the board of pharmacy. The persons so appointed shall hold their offices for five years: *Provided*, That the term of office of the five first appointed shall be so arranged that the term of one shall expire on a given day of each year, and the vacancies so created, as well as all vacancies otherwise occurring, shall be refilled by the governor.

SEC. 7. The said board shall, within thirty days of its appointment, meet and organize by electing a president and secretary from among their members. It shall be the duty of the board to examine all applications for registration submitted in proper form; to grant certificates of registration to such persons as may be entitled to the same under the provisions of this act; to cause the prosecution of all persons violating its provisions; to report annually to the governor the condition of pharmacy in this Territory, which said report shall also furnish a record of the proceedings of the said board for the year and account for all moneys received and disbursed pursuant to this act, and also the names of all pharmacists duly registered under this act. The board shall hold meetings for examination of applicants for registration, and the transaction of such other business as shall pertain to its duties, at least once in three months, and it shall give at least thirty days' public notice of the time of such meetings, shall have power to make by-laws for the proper fulfillment of its duties under this act, and shall keep a book of registration in which shall be entered the names and places of business of all persons registered under this act, which book shall also specify such facts as said person shall claim to justify their registration. Three members of said board shall constitute a quorum.

SEC. 8. Every person applying for registration as registered licentiate or assistant pharmacist shall, before a certificate be granted, pay to the secretary of the board the sum of three dollars, and by every applicant for registration by examination shall be paid the sum of five dollars: *Provided*, That in case of the failure of any applicant to pass a satisfactory examination, his or her money shall be refunded.

SEC. 9. Every registered pharmacist who desires to continue the practice of his profession shall biennially thereafter during the time he shall continue in such practice, on such date as the board of pharmacy may determine, of which date he shall have thirty days' notice by said board, pay to the secretary of the board a registration fee, to be fixed by the board, but which shall in no case exceed two dollars, for which he shall receive a renewal of said registration. The failure of any registered pharmacist to pay said fee shall not deprive him of his right to renewal upon payment thereof; nor shall his retirement from the profession deprive him of the right to renew his registration, should he at any time thereafter wish to resume the practice, upon the payment of said fee. Registered assistants, upon receiving notice as aforesaid, shall, if they desire to renew their registration, pay to the secretary of said board a biennial fee of one dollar. Every certificate of registration granted under this act shall be conspicuously exposed in the pharmacy to which it applies.

SEC. 10. The secretary of the board of pharmacy shall receive a salary, which shall be determined by said board. He shall also receive his traveling and other expenses incurred in the performance of his official duty. The other members of said board shall receive the sum of five dollars for each day actually engaged in such service and all legitimate and necessary expenses incurred in attending the meetings of said board: *Provided,* That no part of the salaries or expenses of the said board shall be paid out of the Territorial treasury. All moneys received in excess of these expenditures shall be held by the secretary of said board as a special fund for meeting future expenses of the board, said secretary giving such bonds as the board shall from time to time direct.

SEC. 11. Any person who is not a registered pharmacist nor licentiate in pharmacy, duly authorized under this act to do business on his own account, who shall, after the expiration of three months from the passage of this act, keep a pharmacy, store, or shop for the dispensing or compounding of physicians' prescriptions, and shall not have in his employ in said pharmacy, store, or shop, a registered pharmacist, nor licentiate in pharmacy, authorized by the Territorial board to manage a pharmacy, shall for each and every offense be liable to a fine of two hundred and fifty dollars.

SEC. 12. Any person not registered under this act who shall take, use, or exhibit the title of registered pharmacist, or licentiate in pharmacy, shall be liable to a fine of one hundred dollars for each and every such offense; a like penalty shall attach to a licentiate in pharmacy who shall, without authority, take, use, or exhibit the title of "registered pharmacist" in the Territory of Utah.

SEC. 13. Any proprietor of a pharmacy, or the person who shall permit the compounding or dispensing of physicians' prescriptions except by a registered pharmacist or licentiate in pharmacy, or under the immediate supervision of one, or who, while continuing in the pursuit of pharmacy in the Territory of Utah, shall fail or neglect to procure his biennial registration, and any person who shall willfully make any false representation to procure, for himself or for another, registration, or shall violate any other provision of this act, shall for each and every such offense be liable to a penalty of one hundred dollars: *Provided,* That nothing in this act shall in any manner interfere with the business of any physician in regular practice, or prevent him from supplying to his patients such articles as may to him seem proper; nor with the business of any dealer except as hereinafter provided: *Provided, also,* That nothing in this act shall in any manner interfere with the business of merchants to sell or vend all such medicines and pharmaceutical preparations as are required by the general public, and bearing the name of the manufacturer.

SEC. 14. The proprietors of all pharmacies shall be held responsible for the quality of all drugs and chemicals sold or dispensed at their respective places of business, except patent and proprietary preparations, and articles sold in the original packages of the manufacturer. Any person who shall willfully adulterate or alter, or cause or permit to be adulterated or altered, any drug, medicine, or pharmaceutical preparation, or shall sell or offer for sale any such adulterated or altered article, and any person who shall substitute one material for another, with the intention to defraud or deceive the purchaser, shall be guilty of a misdemeanor, and liable for prosecution therefor. If convicted he shall pay a fine in any sum less than three hundred dollars for each and every such offense, besides all the cost incurred in investigation and trial. All suits for the recovery of the several penalties prescribed by this act shall be prosecuted in the name of the people of the Territory of Utah in any court of competent jurisdiction; and it shall be the duty of the district attorney, where such offense is committed, to prosecute all persons violating any of the provisions of this act upon proper complaint being made. All penalties collected for such violation shall be paid to the said board of pharmacy, to be held by said board as heretofore directed.

SEC. 15. No such persons shall sell any poisons commonly recognized as such, and especially aconite, arsenic, belladonna, biniodide of mercury, carbolic acid, chloral hydrate, chloroform, conium, corrosive sublimate, creosote, croton oil, cyanide of potassium, digitalis, hydrocyanic acid, laudanum, morphine, nux vomica, oil of bitter almonds, opium, oxalic acid, strychnine, sugar of lead, sulphate of zinc, white precipitate, red precipitate, without affixing to the box, vessel, or package containing the same, and to the wrapper or cover thereof, a red label bearing the name of the article and the word "poison" distinctly shown, with the name and place of business of the seller, who shall not deliver any of said poisons without satisfying himself that said poisons are to be used for legitimate purpose: *Provided*, That nothing herein contained shall apply to the dispensing of physicians' prescriptions of any of the poisons or articles aforesaid. Any person failing to comply with the requirements of this section shall be liable to a fine in any sum less than three hundred dollars for each and every such offense.

SEC. 16. All acts or portions of acts regulating the practice of pharmacy and the sale of poisons within this Territory, enacted prior to the passage of this act, are hereby repealed.

Approved March 10, 1892.

## VERMONT.

Has no pharmacy law.

## VIRGINIA.

### CHAPTER 78, REVISED CODE, 1887.

AN ACT regulating the practice of pharmacy in the State of Virginia.

SECTION 1. The Virginia pharmaceutical association, incorporated by an act of the general assembly approved March third, eighteen hundred and eighty-six, shall continue a corporation under the name of "The Virginia Pharmaceutical Association." Said association shall not hold, at any one time, real estate in excess of ten thousand dollars in value.

SEC. 2. The object of said association is to unite the pharmacists and druggists of this State for mutual aid, encouragement, and improvement; to encourage scientific research, develop pharmaceutical talent, to elevate the standard of professional thought, and ultimately restrict the practice of pharmacy to qualified pharmacists and druggists.

SEC. 3. It shall not be lawful for any person other than a registered pharmacist or practicing physician to retail, compound, or dispense medicines or poisons, or to open or conduct any pharmacy or store for retailing, dispensing, or compounding drugs or medicines, unless such person shall be or shall employ or place in charge of said pharmacy or store a pharmacist registered as hereinafter provided: *Provided*, That nothing herein contained shall prevent the sale by merchants of quinine, Epsom salts, castor oil, essence of peppermint and other flavoring preparations, calomel, camphor, iodide, bromide and chlorate of potassa, opium, paregoric and sweet oil, and such other domestic and proprietary medicines as are usually kept by retail dealers; but the sale of laudanum, morphine, and proprietary medicines must be in original packages as obtained from druggists.

SEC. 4. Any person, in order to be registered, shall be a graduate of some college of pharmacy recognized by the Virginia pharmaceutical association or shall have had three years' experience in a drug store where the prescriptions of medical practitioners are compounded, or shall be a licentiate of pharmacy of the board of pharmacy of Virginia.

SEC. 5. The board of pharmacy of the State of Virginia shall be continued. It shall consist of five members, to be appointed by the governor, each for the term of five years. Their terms of office shall continue to be so arranged that one of them shall go out of office every year. The Virginia pharmaceutical association shall annually recommend five pharmacists, from whom the governor shall select and appoint one to fill the vacancy thus annually occurring in the board. In case of death, resignation, or removal of any member of the board from the State the governor shall, from the names last submitted to him, appoint a pharmacist in his place to serve as a member of the board for the remainder of the term.

SEC. 6. Every person appointed a member of the board shall, before entering upon the duties of his office, take the oath of office in the county or corporation in which he resides, before some officer authorized to administer an oath, and file the certificate of said oath with the board. There shall be a president and secretary of the board, who shall be elected by the board. The term of office of the secretary shall be five years. The board shall hold annual meetings and such other meetings, from time to time, as the business of the board may require. The secretary shall give to each member at least ten days' notice of the time and place of each meeting. Three members shall be a quorum.

SEC. 7. The board shall have authority to transact all business relating to the legal practice of pharmacy; to examine into all cases of abuse, fraud, adulteration, substitution, or malpractice, and to report all violations of this chapter, whenever the same may occur, to the proper State authorities and to said association. It shall be the duty of the board to examine all persons applying for examination in proper form, and to register such as shall establish their rights to registration in accordance with the provisions of this chapter. Anyone examined by the board shall pay a fee of five dollars. In case of failure to pass a satisfactory examination he may be granted a second examination without the payment of a further fee.

SEC. 8. Pharmacists claiming the right of registration under this chapter on account of practical experience shall show to the satisfaction of the said board that they have had not less than three years' practical experience in the preparation of physicians' prescriptions and in compounding and vending medicines and poisons: *Provided*, Nothing in this section shall apply to any person in business on his own account on the 3rd of March, 1886. Licentiates in pharmacy must have had not less than three years' experience previous to the said time in stores where prescriptions of medical practitioners have been prepared, or shall have passed an examination before the board of pharmacy of the State; and in all cases two years shall be required. The board may register, without further examination, the licentiates of such other boards of pharmacy as they may deem proper.

SEC. 9. It shall be the duty of the secretary of the board to keep a book of registration at some convenient place, of which due notice shall be given through the public press, in which shall be entered, under the supervision of the board, the names and the places of business of all persons coming under the provisions of this chapter, and a statement, to be signed by the person making the application, of such facts in the case as he may claim to justify his application. The fee for registration of proprietors shall not exceed two dollars, and for those in the employ of others shall not exceed one dollar. The secretary shall give receipts for all moneys received by him, which moneys shall be used for the purpose of defraying the expenses of the board, and any surplus shall be for the benefit of the association. The salary of the secretary shall be fixed by the board, and paid out of the fees for examination and registration. Each member of the board shall receive the sum of five dollars for every day he is engaged in the services of the board and such actual expenses as may be incurred in going to and from the place of meeting. It shall be the duty of the board, and each member of the association, to report all complaints of non-compliance with or violations of the provisions of this chapter to the proper prosecuting officers of the Commonwealth and to the association; and it shall be the duty of every such officer to prosecute the same when brought to his attention, and there appears to be reasonable grounds for such complaint. The board shall have power to make such rules and regulations as it shall find necessary for carrying into effect the provisions of this chapter, not inconsistent with the purposes and spirit of the same and with the constitution and laws of the State.

SEC. 10. Every person shall be held responsible for the quality of all drugs, chemicals, and medicines he may lawfully sell or dispense with the exception of those sold in the original packages of the manufacturers or taken from the original packages, and also those known as patent medicines, and the essence of lemon, peppermint, and cinnamon, put up for sale for flavoring purposes; and should he intentionally adulterate, or cause to be adulterated, or expose to sale, knowing the same to be adulterated, any of such drugs, chemicals, or medicinal preparations he shall be deemed guilty of misdemeanor, and upon conviction thereof be fined not exceeding one hundred dollars, and in addition thereto, if he be a registered pharmacist, his name may be stricken from the register. Every registered pharmacist who desires to continue the practice of his profession shall annually, within thirty days next preceding the annual meeting of the board, pay to the secretary a registration fee of one dollar, for which he shall receive a renewal of said certificate of registration. Any registered pharmacist failing to renew his registration, as required by this section, and continuing in the exercise of his profession, shall be deemed guilty of misdemeanor, and upon conviction thereof be fined not exceeding twenty-five dollars for each offence.

SEC. 11. It shall not be lawful for any person having authority to sell or dispense medicines or poison to retail any poisons enumerated in the following schedules, without distinctly labeling the bottle, box, vessel, or paper in which said poison is contained, with the name of the article, the word "poison," and the name and place of the business of the seller, to wit:

### SCHEDULE A.

Arsenic, and its preparations, corrosive sublimate, white precipitate, biniodide of mercury, cyanide of potassium, hydrocyanic acid, strychnine, and essential oil of bitter almonds.

### SCHEDULE B.

Aconite, belladonna, colchicum, conium, nux vomica, henbane, savin, ergot, cotton root, cantharides, creosote, digitalis, and their pharmaceutical preparations; croton oil, chloroform, chloral hydrate, sulphate of zinc, carbolic acid, oxalic acid, morphine, preparations containing opium, except paregoric and other preparations of opium containing less than two grains to the ounce, and other deadly poisons. Nor shall it be lawful for any person to sell or deliver any poison mentioned in said schedules unless upon due inquiry it be found that the purchaser is aware of its poisonous nature and represents that it is to be used for a legitimate purpose; nor shall it be lawful for any person to sell any poison mentioned in schedule A without, before delivering the same to the purchaser, causing an entry to be made in a book to be kept for that purpose, always open for public inspection, stating the date of sale, the name and address of the purchaser, the name and quantity of the poison sold, the purpose for which it is required, as represented by the purchaser, and the name of the dispenser. The provisions of this section shall not apply to the dispensing of poisons in usual doses on physicians' prescriptions, put up by a registered pharmacist, or dispensed by a physician.

SEC. 12. Nothing contained in the foregoing section shall apply to or interfere with the business of any practitioner of medicine who does not keep open shop for the retailing of medicines and poisons, nor with the business of wholesale dealers.

SEC. 13. Any person who knowingly or negligently allows the compounding and dispensing of prescriptions in his store or place of business by any person not registered, except under the immediate supervision or control of a registered pharmacist; any person who fraudulently represents himself to be registered; any person not registered who keeps open shop for the retailing or dispensings of medicines or poisons, and any person violating any of the provisions of section seventeen hundred and sixty-four, shall be deemed guilty of misdemeanor, and, on conviction thereof, be fined not less than twenty nor more than one hundred dollars.

## WASHINGTON.

SESSION LAWS OF 1891, CHAPTER 163, TO REGULATE THE PRACTICE OF PHARMACY.

AN ACT to regulate the practice of pharmacy, the licensing of persons to carry on such practice, and the sale of poisons in the State of Washington.

*Be it enacted by the Legislature of the State of Washington:*

SECTION 1. That it shall hereafter be unlawful for any person other than a registered pharmacist to retail, compound, or dispense drugs, medicines, or poisons, or to institute any pharmacy, store, or shop for retailing, compounding, or dispensing drugs, medicines, or poisons, unless such person shall be a registered pharmacist, or shall place in charge of said store a registered pharmacist, except as hereinafter provided.

SEC. 2. In order to be registered, all persons must be either graduates in pharmacy, or shall, at the time this act takes effect, be engaged in the business of a dispensing pharmacist on their own account in the State of Washington, the preparation of physicians' prescriptions, and the vending and compounding of drugs, medicines, and poisons, or shall be licentiates in pharmacy.

SEC. 3. Graduates in pharmacy shall be considered to consist of such persons as have had four years' practical experience in drug stores where prescriptions of medical practitioners are compounded, and have obtained a diploma from such college or schools of pharmacy as shall be approved by the board of pharmacy, as sufficient guarantee of their attainment and proficiency.

SEC. 4. Licentiates in pharmacy shall be such persons as shall have had three years' practical experience in drug stores wherein the prescriptions of medical practitioners are compounded, and have sustained a satisfactory examination before the State board of pharmacy hereinafter mentioned. The State board may grant certificates of registration to licentiates of such other State boards as it may deem proper, without further examination.

SEC. 5. As soon as this act shall take effect the Washington State pharmaceutical association shall elect fifteen reputable and practicing pharmacists doing business in the State, from which the governor shall appoint five. The said five pharmacists, duly elected and appointed, shall constitute the board of pharmacy of the State of Washington, and shall hold office, as respectively designated in their appointments, for the term of one, two, three, four, or five years, as hereinafter provided, and until their successors have been duly elected and appointed. The Washington State pharmaceutical association shall annually elect five pharmacists, from which number the governor of the State shall appoint one to fill [the] vacancy annually occurring in said board. The term of office shall be five years. In case of [a] vacancy occurring from any cause, the governor shall fill the vacancy by appointing a pharmacist, from the names submitted, to serve as a member of the board for the remainder of the term.

SEC. 6. The State board shall, within thirty days after the appointment, meet and organize by the selection of a president and secretary from the number of its own members, who shall be elected for the term of one year, and shall perform the duties prescribed by the board. It shall be the duty of the board to examine all applicants for registration submitted in the proper form ; to grant certificates of registration to such persons as may be entitled to same under the provisions of this act ; to cause prosecutions of all persons violating its provisions ; to report annually to the governor and to the Washington State pharmaceutical association upon the condition of pharmacy in the State, which said report shall also furnish a record of the proceedings of said board for the year, as well as all pharmacists duly registered under this act. The board shall hold meetings for the transaction of such business as shall pertain to its duties once in three months ; and the said board shall give 20 days' public notice of the time and place of such meeting. The said board shall also have power to make by-laws for the proper execution of its duties under this act, and shall keep a book of registration in which shall be entered the names and places of business of all persons registered under this act, also stating facts claimed to justify their registration. Three members of said board shall constitute a quorum.

SEC. 7. Every person claiming the right of registration under this act, who shall, within sixty days after this act takes effect, forward to the board of pharmacy satisfactory proof, supported by his affidavit, that he was engaged in the business of a dispensing pharmacist on his own account in the State of Washington at the time of the passage of this act, as provided in section 2, shall, upon payment of the fee hereinafter mentioned, be granted a certificate of registration: *Provided*, That in case of failure to register as herein specified, then such person shall, in order to be registered, comply with the requirements provided for registration as graduates of pharmacy or licentiates of pharmacy.

SEC. 8. Any person engaged in the position of assistant in pharmacy at the time this act takes effect, not less than eighteen years of age, who shall have had at least three years of practical experience in drug stores where the prescriptions of medical practitioners are compounded, and shall furnish satisfactory evidence to the State board of pharmacy, shall, upon making application for registration and upon payment of $2 to the secretary of said board, within sixty days after this act takes effect, be entitled to a certificate as registered assistant, which certificate shall entitle him to a continuance in such duties as clerk or assistant, but shall not entitle him to engage in business on his own account. Thereafter he shall pay annually to the said secretary the sum of one dollar during the time he shall continue in such duties, in return for which sum he shall receive a renewal of said certificate: *Provided*, Any applicant who has had seven years' experience in compounding medicine immediately prior to the passage of this act may receive a certificate of registered pharmacist.

SEC. 9. Every person claiming registration as a registered pharmacist under section 7 of this act shall, before a certificate is granted, pay to the secretary of the State board of pharmacy the sum of three dollars, and a like sum shall be paid such secretary by graduates in pharmacy, and by such licentiates of other boards who shall apply for registration under this act, and every applicant for registration by examination shall pay to said secretary the sum of five dollars before such examination be attempted: *Provided*, That in case the applicant fail to pass a satisfactory examination, the money shall be held to his credit for a second examination at any time within a year.

SEC. 10. Every registered pharmacist, during the times he continues such practice of his profession, shall annually, on such date as the board of pharmacy may determine, pay to the said secretary of said board of registration a fee of two dollars, in return for which payment he shall receive a renewal of said registration. Every certificate and every renewal shall be conspicuously displayed in the pharmacy to which it applies.

SEC. 11. The secretary of the board of pharmacy shall receive a salary, which salary shall be determined by said board; he shall also receive his traveling and other expenses incurred in the performance of his official duties. The other members of said board shall receive the sum of five dollars for each day actually engaged in such service, and all legitimate and necessary expenses incurred in attending the meetings of said board. Said expenses shall be paid from the fees and penalties received by said board under the provisions of this act, and no part of the salary or other expenses of said board, under the provisions of this act, shall be paid out of the public treasury. All moneys received by said board in excess of said allowance and other expenses hereinbefore provided for shall be held by the secretary of the said board as a special fund for meeting the expenses of said board, said secretary giving such bond as the said board shall, from time to time, direct. The said board shall, in its annual report to the governor and to the Washington State pharmaceutical association, render an account of all money received and disbursed by them pursuant to this act.

SEC. 12. The proprietor of every drug store shall keep in his place of business a registry book in which shall be entered an accurate record of the sales of all mineral acids, carbolic acid, oxalic acid, hydrocyanic acid, cyanide of potassa, arsenic and its preparations, corrosive sublimate, red precipitate, preparations of opium (except paregoric), phosphorus, nux vomica, and strychnine, aconite, belladonna, hellebore, and their preparations, croton oil, oil savin, oil tansy, creosote, wines, and spirituous malt liquors. Said record shall state amount purchased, the date, for what purpose used, buyer's name and address, and said record shall at all times during business hours be subject to the inspection of the prosecuting attorney or to any authorized agent of the board of pharmacy: *Provided*, That no such wines, spirituous, or malt liquors shall be sold for other than medical, scientific, mechanical, or sacramental purposes. Furthermore, that all poisons shall be plainly labeled as such, and that such labels shall also bear the name and address of the druggist selling the same. The provisions of this section shall not apply to dispensing by physicians' prescriptions.

SEC. 13. Any person not being a registered pharmacist within the full meaning of this act who shall, after the expiration of sixty days from the time this act shall take effect, retail, compound, or dispense medicines, or who shall take, use, or exhibit the title of registered pharmacist shall, for each and every said offense, be liable to a penalty of fifty dollars. Any registered pharmacist or other person who shall permit the compounding and dispensing of prescriptions or the vending of drugs, medicines, or poisons in his store or place of business, except under the supervision of a registered pharmacist, or except by a registered assistant, or any pharmacist or registered assistant who, while continuing in business, shall fail or neglect to procure his annual registration, or any person who shall willfully make any false representations to procure registration for himself or any other person, or who shall violate any of the provisions of this act shall, for each and every offense, be liable to a penalty of fifty dollars: *Provided*, That nothing in this act shall in any manner interfere with the business of any physician in regular practice, or prevent him from supplying to his patients such articles as he may deem proper, nor with the making of proprietary medicine or medicines placed in sealed packages, nor prevent shopkeepers from dealing in and selling the commonly used medicines and poisons, if such medicines and poisons are put up by a registered pharmacist, nor with the exclusive wholesale business of any dealers, except as heretofore provided.

SEC. 14. Every proprietor of a drug store shall be held responsible for the quality of all drugs, chemicals, or medicines sold or dispensed by him, except those sold in original packages of the manufacturer, and except those articles or preparations known as patent or proprietary medicine.

SEC. 15. Any person who shall knowingly, willfully, or fraudulently falsify or adulterate any drug or medical substance, or any preparation authorized or recognized by the Pharmacopœia of the United States, or used or intended to be used in medical practice, or shall willingly, knowingly, or fraudulently sell or cause the same to be sold for medical purposes, shall be deemed guilty of a misdemeanor, and upon conviction shall pay a penalty not exceeding $500.00, and shall forfeit to the State of Washington all articles so adulterated.

SEC. 16. All suits for the recovery of the several penalties prescribed in this act shall be prosecuted in the name of the State of Washington in any court having jurisdiction, and it shall be the duty of the prosecuting attorney of the county wherein such offense is committed to prosecute all persons violating the provisions of this act, upon proper complaint being made. All penalties collected under the provisions of this act shall inure one-half to the State board of pharmacy and one-half to the school fund of the county in which suit was prosecuted and judgment obtained.

SEC. 17. All acts or portions of acts regulating the practice of pharmacy or adulteration of drugs within this State in conflict with this act are hereby repealed.

Approved, March 9, 1891.

# 141

## WEST VIRGINIA.

AN ACT to regulate the practice of pharmacy and the sale of medicines and poisons.

[Chapter 52, passed February 21, 1881, as amended and reënacted by chapter 112 of the acts 1882, adjourned session, passed March 25, 1882.]

*Be it enacted by the Legislature of West Virginia:*

SECTION 1. It shall be unlawful for any person not a registered pharmacist or who does not employ as his salesman a registered pharmacist within the meaning of this act, to conduct any pharmacy, drug store, apothecary shop, or store for the purpose of retailing, compounding, or dispensing medicines or poisons for medical use, except as hereinafter provided.

SEC. 2. It shall be unlawful for the proprietor of any store or pharmacy to allow any person except a registered pharmacist to compound or dispense the prescriptions of physicians, or to retail or dispense the poisons named in schedules A and B herein, for medical use, except as an aid to or under the supervision of a registered pharmacist.

SEC. 3. The board of public works shall appoint one person from each Congressional district from among the most competent pharmacists of the State, all of whom shall have been residents of the State for five years and of at least five years' practical experience in their profession, who shall be known as "commissioners of pharmacy for the State of West Virginia;" one of whom shall hold his office for one year, one for two years, one for three years, and one for four years, and each until his successor shall be appointed and qualified; and each year thereafter one commissioner shall be so appointed for four years and until a successor be appointed and qualified. If a vacancy occur in said commission, another shall be appointed, as aforesaid, to fill the unexpired term thereof. Said commissioners, a majority of whom may act, shall have power to make by-laws and all necessary regulations for the proper fulfillment of their duties under this act, without expense to the State, and to examine applicants and grant certificates.

SEC. 4. The commissioners of pharmacy shall register, in a suitable book, a duplicate of which is to be kept in the office of the secretary of state, the names and place of business of all persons to whom they issue certificates, and the dates thereof. It shall be the duty of said commissioners of pharmacy to register, without examination, as registered pharmacists, all pharmacists and druggists who are engaged in business in the State of West Virginia at the passage of this act as owners or principals of stores or pharmacies for selling at retail, compounding, or dispensing drugs, medicines, or chemicals for medical use, or for compounding and dispensing physicians' prescriptions; and all assistant pharmacists, not under eighteen years of age, engaged in said stores or pharmacies in the State of West Virginia at the passage of this act, and who have been engaged as such in some store or pharmacy where physicians' prescriptions were compounded and dispensed for not less than five years prior to the passage of this act: *Provided, however,* That in case of failure or neglect on the part of such person or persons to apply for registration within sixty days after they shall have been notified, they shall undergo an examination such as is provided for in section five of this act.

SEC. 5. That the said commissioners of pharmacy shall, upon application, and at such time and place and in such manner as they may determine, examine, orally or otherwise, under such regulations as they may by by-law prescribe, each and every person who shall desire to conduct the business of selling at retail, compounding or dispensing drugs, medicines, or chemicals for medicinal use, or compounding or dispensing physicians' prescriptions as pharmacists. And if a majority of said commissioners shall be satisfied that said person is competent and fully qualified to conduct said business of compounding or dispensing drugs, medicines, or chemicals for medicinal use, or to compound or dispense physicians' prescriptions, they shall enter the name of such person as a registered pharmacist in the book provided for in section four of this act; and that all graduates in pharmacy having a diploma from an incorporated college or school of pharmacy that requires a practical experience in pharmacy of not less than four years before granting a diploma, shall be entitled to have their names registered as pharmacist by said commissioners of pharmacy without examination.

SEC. 6. That the commissioners of pharmacy shall be entitled to demand and receive from each person whom they register and furnish a certificate as a registered pharmacist, without examination, the sum of two dollars, and from each and every person whom they examine orally or otherwise, the sum of five dollars, which shall be in full for services. And in case the said examination of said person shall prove defective and unsatisfactory and his name not be registered, he shall be permitted to present himself for reexamination within any period not exceeding twelve months next thereafter, and no charge shall be made for such reexamination.

SEC. 7. Every applicant for registration as a pharmacist shall present to the commissioners of pharmacy satisfactory evidence that he is a person of good moral character and not addicted to drunkenness, and all persons, whether registered pharmacists or not, shall be held responsible for the quality of all drugs, chemicals, and medicines they may sell or dispense, with the exception of those sold in the original packages of the manufacturer, and those known as "patent medicines." Any person who shall knowingly, intentionally, and fraudulently adulterate or cause to be adulterated any drugs, chemicals, or medical preparations, or knowingly sell any adulterated drugs, chemicals, or medical preparations, shall be deemed guilty of a misdemeanor, and upon conviction thereof be fined not exceeding one hundred dollars, and if he be a registered pharmacist his name shall be stricken from the register.

SEC. 8. Apothecaries registered as in this act provided, shall have the right to keep and sell, under such restrictions as herein provided, all medicines and poisons, authorized by the national, American, or United States dispensatory and pharmacopœia, as of recognized utility.

SEC. 9. No druggist or registered pharmacist shall retail any of the poisons enumerated in the following schedule except as hereinafter provided.

SCHEDULE A.

Arsenic and its preparations, corrosive sublimate, white precipitate, red precipitate, biniodide of mercury, cyanide of potassium, hydrocyanic acid, strychnia, and all other poisonous vegetable alkaloids and their salts; essential oil of bitter almonds, opium and its preparations, except paregoric and other preparations of opium containing less than two grains to the ounce.

SCHEDULE B.

Aconite, belladonna, colchicum, conium, nux vomica, henbene, savin, ergot, cotton root, cantharides, creosote, digitalis, and their pharmaceutical preparations; croton oil, chloroform, chloral hydrate, sulphate of zinc, sulphate of copper, acetate of lead, mineral acids, carbolic acid, and oxalic acid.

Whenever any of the said poisons are sold, the box, vessel, or paper, in which the same is put up shall be distinctly labeled with a device bearing the death's head and crossbones, and also the name of the article, the word "poison," and the name and place of business of seller. The seller shall also ascertain upon due inquiry that the purchaser is aware of the poisonous character of the drug, and that it is to be used for a legitimate and lawful purpose. He shall also, before delivering any of the poisons named in schedule A to a purchaser, cause an entry to be made in a book kept for the purpose, which entry shall show the date of the sale, the name and residence of the purchaser, the name and quality of the poison sold, the purpose for which it is to be used as represented by the purchaser, and the name of the dispenser; such book to be always subject to the inspection of the proper authorities, and to be preserved for at least five years from the date of the last entry.

The provisions of this section shall not apply to the dispensing of drugs in not unusual quantities on the prescriptions of physicians.

Nothing in this act contained shall be construed so as to protect any druggist or registered pharmacist from any penalty or forfeiture prescribed in any other law regulating the sale of alcoholic or other intoxicating liquors; and the name of any registered pharmacist who shall be convicted twice of the violation of such law shall be stricken from the register and he shall no longer be a registerd pharmacist. Nor shall this act be construed to authorize any person to carry on the business of a druggist without having first obtained a license therefor, if such license be required by any other law, or to sell, offer, or expose for sale any of the liquors, drinks, mixtures, or preparations mentioned in section 1 of chapter 32 of the Code of West Virginia, as amended and reenacted by chapter 107 of the Acts of 1877, except for medicinal, mechanical, or scientific purposes. And if any person carrying on or interested in the business of a druggist shall, in violation of this section, sell any such liquors, drinks, mixtures, or preparations he shall be guilty of a misdemeanor, and for each offense be fined not less than twenty-five nor more than one hundred dollars; and it shall be the special duty of the judge of every circuit court to give this provision in charge to the grand juries of their respective courts. In any prosecution against a person carrying on or interested in the business of a druggist for selling any such liquors, drinks, mixtures, or preparations, contrary to law, if the sale be proved, it shall be presumed that such sale was unlawful unless the contrary be shown.

SEC. 10. No person shall procure, or attempt to procure, registration for himself, or for another, under this act, by making, or causing to be made, any false representations, nor shall any person not a registered pharmacist, as provided in this act, conduct a store, pharmacy, or place for retailing, compounding, or dispensing drugs, medicines, or chemicals for medicinal use, or for compounding or dispensing physicians' prescriptions, or take, use, or exhibit the title of a registered pharmacist.

SEC. 11. This act shall not apply to physicians putting up their own prescriptions, nor to anyone not doing business in an incorporated city or town who sells such ordinary drugs as are usually kept in country stores, nor to such person in any such city or town in which there is no registered pharmacist engaged in the business of selling drugs; but the term ordinary drugs shall not be held to include any of the poisons named in schedules A and B, nor any intoxicating liquor.

SEC. 12. It shall be the duty of the board to investigate all complaints and charges of noncompliance or violation of the provisions of this act, and to bring the same to the notice of the proper prosecuting officer, as provided for in section seven of this act, whenever there appears to the board reasonable grounds for such action.

SEC. 13. Every registered pharmacist shall keep his certificate of registration posted in a conspicuous place at his place of business, and any failure so to do shall be deemed and held to be *prima facie* evidence that such person is not a registered pharmacist.

SEC. 14. Any person violating any of the provisions of this act shall be guilty of a misdemeanor, and for every such offense shall be fined not less than twenty-five nor more than one hundred dollars, and (except as provided in section seven of this act) the name of any person convicted of such violation shall be stricken from the register and he shall no longer be a registered pharmacist in this State.

It shall be the duty of the clerk of the court in which, or the justice of the peace before whom, any conviction is had to transmit forthwith a certified copy of the record entry of such conviction to the commissioners of pharmacy, who shall thereupon strike the name of the person so convicted from the register.

All fines collected under any of the provisions of this act shall be paid one-half to the State school fund and the other half to the commissioners of pharmacy.

## ACTS REPEALED.

All acts and parts of acts coming within the purview of this act, and inconsistent therewith, are hereby repealed.

Passed March 25, 1882. Approved March 28, 1882.

[Note by the clerk of the house of delegates.]

The foregoing act takes effect from its passsage, two-thirds of the members elected to each house, by a vote taken by yeas and nays, having so directed.

A true copy from the rolls.

Attest:

J. B. PEYTON,
*Clerk of the House of Delegates and Keeper of the Rolls.*

## WISCONSIN.

### CHAPTER 167, LAWS OF 1882, AS AMENDED IN 1885 AND 1887.

AN ACT to regulate the practice of pharmacy, the licensing of persons to carry on such practice, and the sale of poisons in the State of Wisconsin.

*The people of the State of Wisconsin, represented in Senate and Assembly, do enact as follows:*

SECTION 1 (as amended by chapter 146, Laws of 1885). That it shall hereafter be unlawful for any person other than a registered pharmacist to retail, compound, or dispense drugs, medicines ...sons (except Paris green, when kept in stock, put up in pound and half-pou... ...ages), or to institute or conduct any pharmacy, store, or shop for retailing, ...ding, or dispensing drugs, medicines, or poisons, unless such person shall b.. ...istered p' armacist, or shall employ and place in charge of such pharmacy, ...re or shop.. ,egistered pharmacist within the full meaning of this act, excep.. as hereinafter provided.

SEC. 2. In order to be registered within the full meaning of this act all persons must be either graduates in pharmacy, or shall at the time this act takes effect be engaged in the business of a dispensing pharmacist on their own account, in the State of Wisconsin, in the proper tion of physicians' prescriptions, and in the vending and compounding of drugs, medicines, and poisons, or shall be licentiates in pharmacy.

SEC. 3. Graduates in pharmacy shall be considered to consist of such persons as have had four years' practical experience in drug stores where prescriptions of medical practitioners are compounded, and have obtained a diploma from such colleges or schools of pharmacy as shall be approved by the board of pharmacy, such as shall be judged by the said board of pharmacy as sufficient guarantee of their attainments and proficiency.

SEC. 4 (as amended by chapter 460, Laws of 1887). Licentiates in pharmacy shall be such persons as shall have had five years' practical experience in drug stores wherein prescriptions of medical practitioners are compounded and have sustained a satisfactory examination before the State board of pharmacy hereinafter mentioned. The State board may grant certificates of registration to licentiates of such other State boards as it may deem proper without further examination. It shall be the duty of the said board to grant an assistant's certificate to such persons as have had two years' practical experience in drug stores where prescriptions of medical practitioners are compounded and have passed a satisfactory examination before said board of pharmacy. The holder of such assistant's certificate shall, however, be deemed competent to sell, vend, and compound on his own account such medicines as are required by the general public in towns or villages having less than five hundred inhabitants.

SEC. 5. Immediately upon the passage of this act the Wisconsin pharmaceutical association shall elect ten reputable and practicing pharmacists doing business in the State, from which number the governor of the State shall appoint five. The said five pharmacists, duly elected and appointed, shall constitute the board of pharmacy of the State of Wisconsin, and shall hold office, as respectively designated in their appointments, for the term of one, two, three, four, and five years, respectively, as hereinafter provided, and until their successors have been duly appointed and qualified. The Wisconsin pharmaceutical society shall annually thereafter elect three pharmacists, from which number the governor of the State shall appoint one to fill the vacancy annually occurring in said board. The term of office shall be five years. In case of resignation or removal from the State of any member of said board, or of a vacancy occurring from any cause, the governor shall fill the vacancy by appointing a pharmacist from the names last submitted, to serve as a member of the board for the remainder of the term.

SEC. 6. The said board shall, within thirty days of its appointment, meet and organize by the selection of a president and secretary from the number of its own members, who shall be elected for the term of one year, and shall perform the duties prescribed by the board. It shall be the duty of the board to examine all applications for registration submitted in proper form; to grant certificates of registration to such persons as may be entitled to the same under the provisions of this act; to cause the prosecution of all persons violating its provisions; to report annually to the governor and to the Wisconsin pharmaceutical society upon the condition of pharmacy in the State, which said report shall also furnish a record of the proceedings of said board for the year, as well as the names of all pharmacists duly registered under this act. The board shall hold meetings for the examination of applicants for registration and the transaction of such other business as shall pertain to its duties at least once in three months; and the State board shall give thirty days' public notice of the time and place of such meeting. The said board shall also have power to make by-laws for the proper execution of its duties under this act, and shall keep a book of registration, in which shall be entered the names and places of business of all persons registered under this act, which registration book shall also contain such facts as said persons shall claim to justify their registration. Three members of said board shall constitute a quorum.

SEC. 7. Every person claiming the right of registration under this act who shall, within three months after the passage of this act, forward to the board of pharmacy satisfactory proof, supported by his affidavit, that he was engaged in the business of dispensing pharmacist on his own account in the State of Wisconsin at the time of the passage of this act, as provided in section 2, shall, upon the payment of the fee hereinafter mentioned, be granted a certificate of registration : *Provided,* That in case of failure or neglect to register as herein specified then such person shall, in order to be registered, comply with the requirements provided for registration as graduates in pharmacy or licentiates in pharmacy within the meaning of this act.

SEC. 8. Any person engaged in the position of assistant or clerk in a pharmacy at the time this act takes effect, no less than eighteen years of age, who shall have had at least two years' practical experience in drug stores where the prescriptions of medical practitioners are compounded and who shall furnish satisfactory evidence to that effect to the State board of pharmacy, shall, upon making application for registration and upon payment to the secretary of said board of a fee of one dollar, within sixty days after this act takes effect, be entitled to a certificate as "registered assistant," which certificate shall entitle him to continue in such duties as clerk or assistant; but such certificate shall not entitle him to engage in business on his own account, except as provided in section 4, or to the certificate of registered pharmacist, unless he shall have had at least five years' experience in such stores where the prescriptions of medical practitioners are compounded at the time of the passage of this act. Thereafter he shall pay annually to the said secretary a sum not exceeding fifty cents, during the time he shall continue in such duties, in return for which sum he shall receive a renewal of his certificate.

SEC. 9. Every person claiming registration as a registered pharmacist under section 7 of this act shall, before a certificate is granted, pay to the secretary of said board of pharmacy the sum of two dollars, and a like sum shall be paid to said secretary by graduates in pharmacy and by such licentiates of other boards who shall apply for registration under this act; and every applicant for registration by examination shall pay to the said secretary the sum of five dollars before such examination be attempted: *Provided*, That if the applicant fails to sustain a satisfactory examination by the said board his money, the said five dollars, shall be refunded to him.

SEC. 10, as amended by chapter 460, laws of 1887. Every registered pharmacist who desires to continue the practice of his profession shall annually, during the time he shall continue such practice, on such date as the board of pharmacy may determine, pay to the secretary of said board a registration fee, the amount of which shall be fixed by the board, and which in no case shall exceed two dollars in return for which payment he shall receive a renewal of said registration. Every certificate of registration and every renewal of such certificate shall be conspicuously exposed in the pharmacy to which it applies, and if any registered pharmacist or assistant pharmacist shall fail or neglect to conspicuously expose such certificate he shall be fined not less than five dollars and not more than ten dollars and costs for each and every offense.

SEC. 11. The secretary of the board of pharmacy shall receive a salary which shall be determined by said board; he shall also receive his traveling and other expenses incurred in the performance of his official duties. The other members of said board shall receive the sum of five dollars for each day actually engaged in such service and all legitimate and necessary expenses incurred in attending the meetings of said board. Said expenses shall be paid from the fees and penalties received by said board under the provisions of this act; and no part of the salary or other expenses of said board shall be paid out of the public treasury. All moneys received by said board in excess of said allowances and other expenses hereinbefore provided for, shall be held by the secretary of said board as a special fund for meeting the expenses of said board, said secretary giving such bonds as the said board shall from time to time direct. The said board shall, in its annual report to the governor and to the Wisconsin pharmaceutical association, render an account of all moneys received and disbursed by them pursuant to this act.

SEC. 12, as amended by chapter 460, laws of 1887. Any member not being or not having in his employ a registered pharmacist, within the full meaning of this act, except as provided in section 4, who shall, after the expiration of ninety days from the passage of this act, keep a pharmacy store or shop for retailing, compounding, or dispensing medicines, or who shall take, use, or exhibit the title of a registered pharmacist, shall, for each and every offense, be liable to a penalty of fifty dollars. Any registered pharmacist or any person who shall permit the compounding and dispensing of prescriptions or the vending of drugs, medicines, or poisons in his store or place of business, except under the personal supervision of a registered pharmacist, or except by a registered assistant pharmacist, or any pharmacist or "registered assistant," who, while continuing in business, shall fail or neglect to procure his annual registration, or any person who shall willfully make any false representation to procure registration for himself or any other person, or who shall violate any other provision of this act, shall, for each and every such offense, be liable to a penalty of fifty dollars: *Provided*, That nothing in this act shall in any manner interfere with the business of any physician in regular practice, or prevent him from supplying to his patients such articles as may seem to him proper, nor with the making and vending of proprietary medicine or medicines placed in sealed packages, with the name of the contents and of the pharmacist or physician by whom prepared or compounded, nor with the sale of the usual domestic remedies by retail dealers, nor with the exclusively wholesale business of any dealers, except as heretofore provided.

SEC. 13. Every proprietor or conductor of a drug store shall be held responsible for the quality of all drugs, chemicals, and medicines sold or dispensed by him, articles or preparations known as patent or proprietary medicines. And should such proprietor or conductor of a drug store knowingly, intentionally, and fraudulently adulterate or cause to be adulterated such drugs, chemicals, or medical preparations he shall be deemed guilty of a misdemeanor, and upon conviction thereof shall be liable to a penalty of not less than seventy-five dollars nor more than one hundred and fifty dollars, and his name stricken from the register.

SEC. 14. No persons shall sell at retail any poisons commonly recognized as such, and especially aconite, arsenic, belladonna, biniodide of mercury, carbolic acid, chloral hydrate, chloroform, conium, corrosive sublimate, creosote, croton oil, cyanide of potassium, digitalis, hydrocyanic acid, laudanum, morphine, nux vomica, oil of bitter almonds, opium, oxalic acid, strychnine, sugar of lead, sulphate of zinc, white precipitate, red precipitate, without affixing to the box, bottle, vessel, or package containing the same, and to the wrapper or cover thereof, a label bearing the name "poison," distinctly shown, together with the name and place of business of the seller. Nor shall he deliver any of the said poisons to any person without satisfying himself that such poison is to be used for legitimate purposes: *Provided,* That nothing herein contained shall apply to the dispensing of physicians' prescriptions specifying any of the poisons aforesaid. Any person failing to comply with the requirements of this section shall be deemed guilty of a misdemeanor, and shall be liable to a fine of not less than five dollars for each and every such omission.

SEC. 15, as amended by chapter 460, laws of 1887. All suits for the recovery of the several penalties prescribed in this act shall be prosecuted in the name of the State of Wisconsin, in any court having jurisdiction; and it shall be the duty of the district attorney of the county wherein such offense is committed to prosecute all persons violating the provisions of this act upon proper complaint being made. All penalties collected under the provisions of this act shall inure to the school fund of the State.

SEC. 16. All acts or portions of acts regulating the practice of pharmacy and the sale of poisons within this State, enacted prior to the passage of this act, are hereby repealed: *Provided,* That nothing in this act shall be so construed as to prevent any person who has once been a registered member, and may have forfeited his membership by nonpayment of dues or fees, from renewing his membership by paying the required dues or fees without examination.

CHAPTER 296, LAWS OF 1885, AS AMENDED, RELATING TO THE SALE OF POISONS BY PHARMACISTS, ETC.

SEC. 2, as amended by chapter 404, laws of 1887. There is hereby enacted a new section, to be known as section 1548a of the revised statutes, which shall read as follows: Section 1548a. The town boards, village boards, and common councils of the respective towns, villages, and cities in the State, upon the written application of any registered pharmacist, may grant to such registered pharmacist as they deem proper a permit to sell strong, spirituous, and ardent liquors in quantities less than one gallon, for medicinal, mechanical, or scientific purposes only, and not to be drank on the premises. The sum to be paid for such permit shall be ten dollars, and such permit shall be granted and issued in the same manner and terminate at the same time as the license provided for in the preceding section, except that it shall not be necessary for any such registered pharmacist to furnish the bond required by section 1549 of the revised statutes: *Provided,* That in case any town board, village board, or common council shall refuse to grant such permit, any registered pharmacist may sell such strong, spirituous, and ardent liquors, for medicinal purposes only, on the written prescription for each sale of a practicing physician, competent to testify in any court in this State in a professional capacity, as provided by section 1436 of the revised statutes. It shall be the duty of every pharmacist to whom a permit is issued to keep a book, in which he shall enter the date of every sale made by him, of any such liquors, the name of t̶h̶e̶ ̶p̶e̶rson t̶o̶ ̶who̶m̶ ̶s̶o̶l̶d̶ ̶a̶n̶d̶ ̶t̶h̶e̶ purpose for which such liquors are sold; and such book shall at all times be open to the inspection of the authorities granting such permit. It shall be the duty of every such pharmacist, on the third Tuesday of April in each year, to file with the clerk of the city, village, or town in which the permit is granted a verified copy of all the entries made by him in such book, as he is required by this section to keep.

SEC. 5. There is hereby enacted a new section, to be known as section 1550a of the revised statutes, which shall read as follows: Section 1550a. Any person who shall, for the purpose of inducing the sale of liquors by any registered pharmacist, holding a permit therefor, for any other use than medicinal, mechanical, or scientific purposes, make any false statement or representation to such pharmacist, or any clerk or employé of such pharmacist, regarding the use for which such liquor is bought, and thereby induce such sale to be made in violation of law, or any registered pharmacist holding a permit under this chapter, who shall neglect or refuse to comply with any of the requirements of this chapter, shall be guilty of a misdemeanor, and on conviction thereof shall be punished therefor by a fine of not less than ten dollars or more than forty dollars, besides the costs of suit; and in case of a second or any subsequent conviction of the same person, the punishment shall be by a fine of not less than forty dollars or more than one hundred dollars, besides the costs of suit, or by imprisonment, in the county jail of the proper county, not less than thirty days or more than three months; and in case of punishment by fine, such person shall, unless the fine and costs be paid forthwith, be committed to the county jail of the proper county until such fine and costs are paid, or until discharged by due course of law.

FORM OF CERTIFICATE USED IN WISCONSIN.

| | WISCONSIN STATE BOARD OF PHARMACY. | |
|---|---|---|
| CHAS. R. BECHMANN, *President.* | | Place over the signatures on your certificate. |
| | *Registration of certificate No. 520.* | |
| HENRY C. SCHRANCK. | RENEWAL | June 22, 1892. |
| R. D. SURFONTS. | [Wisconsin State Board of Pharmacy. 1882. Seal.] | *For the term of one year, from June 1, A. D. 1892.* |
| F. ROBINSON. | | E. B. HEIMSTREET, *Secretary.* |

Every certificate of registration and every renewal of such certificate shall be conspicuously exposed in the pharmacy to which it applies. (*See* Sec. 10, Pharmacy Law.)

## WYOMING.

AN ACT to regulate the practice of pharmacy in the Territory of Wyoming, and for other purposes.

*Be it enacted by the Council and House of Representatives of the Territory of Wyoming:*

SECTION 1. It shall not be lawful for any person, other than a registered pharmacist, to retail, compound, or dispense drugs, medicines, or poisons, or to open or conduct any pharmacy or store for retailing, compounding, or dispensing drugs, medicines, or poisons unless such person shall be, or shall employ and place in charge of said pharmacy or store, a registered pharmacist within the meaning of this act, except as hereinafter provided.

SEC. 2. Any person, in order to be registered within the meaning of this act, must be a graduate in pharmacy, or a licentiate in pharmacy, or shall be engaged at the time this act takes effect, and shall have been engaged for a period of four years prior thereto, in the business of a dispensing pharmacist on his own account in this

Territory in the preparation of physicians' prescriptions, and in the vending and compounding of drugs, medicines, and poisons.

SEC. 3. Licentiates in pharmacy must be such persons as have had two consecutive years of practical experience in drug stores wherein the prescriptions of medical practitioners are compounded, and have passed a satisfactory examination before commissioners of pharmacy hereinafter mentioned. The commissioners of pharmacy may grant certificates of registration, without further examination, to graduates in pharmacy who have obtained a diploma from such colleges or schools of pharmacy as shall be approved by said commission, and may also grant certificates of registration, without further examination, to the licentiates of such other State or Territorial boards of pharmacy as they may deem proper.

SEC. 4. The governor shall nominate, and by and with the advice and consent of the legislative council, shall appoint three persons from among such competent pharmacists in the Territory as have had five years' practical experience in the dispensing of physicians prescriptions, who shall constitute the commissioners of pharmacy herein named. The persons so appointed shall hold their offices for the term of six years, and until their successors are appointed and qualified: *Provided*, That the term of office of the three commissioners first appointed shall be so arranged that the term of one shall expire on the thirty-first day of March in each second year hereafter, and the vacancies so occurring shall be filled by appointment by the governor, made with the advice and consent of the council. All vacancies occurring during the recess of the legislative council shall be filled in the manner provided by law. The said commissioners shall be appointed from different counties, so as to represent the several portions of the Territory as nearly as practicable.

SEC. 5. The said commission shall, within thirty days after its appointment, meet and organize by the election of a president and secretary from its own numbers, who shall be elected for the term of one year and shall perform the duties prescribed by the commission. It shall be the duty of the commission to examine all applications for registration submitted in proper form; to grant certificates of registration to such persons as may be entitled to the same under the provisions of this act; to cause the prosecution of all persons violating its provisions; to report annually to the governor upon the condition of pharmacy in the Territory, which said report shall also furnish a record of the proceedings of the said commission for the year, and also the names of all pharmacists duly registered under this act. The commission shall hold meetings for the examination of applicants for registration, and the transaction of such other business as shall pertain to its duties, at least once in four months. Said commission shall have power to make by-laws for the proper fulfillment of its duties under this act, and shall keep a book of registration, in which shall be kept the names and places of business of all persons registered under this act, together with the date of registration, which book shall also specify such facts as said persons shall claim to justify their registration. Two members of said commission shall constitute a quorum.

SEC. 6. Every person claiming the right of registration under this act who shall within three months after this act shall take effect, forward to the commissioners of pharmacy satisfactory proof, supported by his affidavit, that he was engaged in the business of a dispensing pharmacist on his own account in this Territory at the time this act takes effect, as provided in section two, shall, upon the payment of the fee hereinafter mentioned, be granted a certificate of registration: *Provided*, That in case of failure or neglect to register, as herein provided, then such person shall, in order to be registered, comply with the requirements provided for registration as a graduate in pharmacy or a licentiate in pharmacy within the meaning of this act.

SEC. 7. Any assistant or clerk in pharmacy who shall not have the qualification of a registered pharmacist within the meaning of this act, not less than eighteen years of age, who at the time this act takes effect shall have been employed or engaged two years or more in drug stores where the prescriptions of medical practitioners are compounded, and shall furnish satisfactory evidence to that effect to the commissioners of pharmacy, shall, upon making application for registration, and upon the payment to the secretary of said commission of a fee of two dollars, within sixty days after this act takes effect, be entitled to a certificate as a "registered assistant," which said certificate shall entitle him to continue in such duties as clerk or assistant; but such certificate shall not entitle him to engage in business on his own account unless he shall have at least five years' experience in pharmacy at the time of the passage of this act. Annually thereafter, during the time he shall continue in such duties, he shall pay to the secretary a sum not exceeding one dollar and a half, for which he shall receive a renewal of his certificate.

SEC. 8. Every person applying for registration as a registered pharmacist under section six of this act shall, before a certificate is granted, pay to the secretary of the commission the sum of three dollars, and a like sum shall be paid to said secretary by graduates in pharmacy, and by licentiates of other commissions who shall apply for registration; and every applicant for registration by examination shall pay the sum of ten dollars to said secretary before examination. If the applicant fails to pass a satisfactory examination his money shall be refunded, and he shall not be eligible for reëxamination within four months from the date of such previous examination. After the said four months have elapsed the applicant shall be entitled to a reëxamination upon the payment of a fee of ten dollars, as aforesaid, but such fee shall not be refunded if the applicant fails to pass a satisfactory examination. Upon failing to satisfactorily pass the second examination the applicant may be reëxamined at any regular meeting of the commission upon the payment of a fee of three dollars.

SEC. 9. Every registered pharmacist who desires to continue the practice of his profession shall annually thereafter, during the time he shall continue in such practice, on such date as the commission of pharmacy may determine, pay to the secretary of the said commission a registered fee, to be fixed by the commission, but which shall in no case exceed two dollars, for which he shall receive a renewal of said registration. Every certificate of registration granted under this act shall be conspicuously exposed in the pharmacy to which it applies. Any registered pharmacist who shall sever his connection with the drug business for a period of three successive years shall not be entitled to renew his registration except upon passing a satisfactory examination, as provided for in this act.

SEC. 10. The secretary of the commission shall receive a salary, which shall be fixed by the commission; he shall also receive his traveling and other expenses incurred in the performance of his official duties. The other members of the commission shall receive the sum of five dollars for each day actually engaged in this service and all legitimate and necessary expenses incurred in attending the meetings of said board. Said expenses shall be paid from the fees and penalties received by the commission under the provisions of this act, and no part of the salary or other expenses of the commission shall be paid out of the Territorial treasury. All moneys received in excess of said per diem allowance and other expenses above provided for shall be held by the secretary as a special fund for meeting the expenses of said commission, he giving such bonds as the commission shall from time to time direct. The commission shall, in its annual report to the governor, render an account of all moneys received and disbursed by them pursuant to this act.

SEC. 11. Any person not being or having in his employ a registered pharmacist within the meaning of this act, who shall, three months after this act takes effect, keep a pharmacy or store for retailing or compounding medicines, or who shall take, use, or exhibit the title of a registered pharmacist, shall, for each and every such offense, be liable to a penalty of fifty dollars. Any registered pharmacist who shall permit the compounding and dispensing of prescriptions or the vending of drugs, medicines, or poisons in his store or place of business, except under the supervision of a registered pharmacist, or except by a "registered assistant" pharmacist, or any pharmacist or "registered assistant" who, while continuing in business, shall fail or neglect to procure his annual registration, or any person who shall willfully make any false representation to procure registration for himself or any other person, shall, for every offense, be liable to a penalty of fifty dollars: *Provided*, That nothing in this act shall apply to nor in any way interfere with the business of any physician or prevent him from supplying to his patients such articles as may seem to him proper, nor with the making or vending of patent or proprietary medicines, or medicines placed in sealed packages, with the name of the contents and of the pharmacist or physician by whom prepared or compounded, nor with the sale of the usual domestic remedies by retail dealers, nor with the exclusively wholesale business of any dealers, as hereinafter provided: *And provided, further,* That no part of this section shall be so construed as to give the right to any physician to furnish any intoxicating liquors as a beverage, on prescription or otherwise.

Sec. 12. No person shall add to or remove from any drug, medicine, chemical, or pharmaceutical preparation any ingredient or material for the purpose of adulteration or substitution, or which shall deteriorate the quality, commercial or medicinal effect, or which shall alter the nature or composition of such drug, medicine, chemical, or pharmaceutical preparation so that it will not correspond to the recognized test of identity or purity. Any person who shall thus willfully adulterate or alter, or cause to be adulterated or altered, or shall sell or offer for sale any such adulterated or altered drug, medicine, chemical, or pharmaceutical preparation, or any person who shall substitute, or cause to be substituted, one material for another with the intention to defraud or deceive the purchaser, shall be guilty of a misdemeanor and be liable to prosecution under this act. If convicted he shall be liable to all the costs of the action and all expenses incurred by the commissioners of pharmacy in connection therewith, and for the first offense be liable to a fine of not less than fifty dollars nor more than one hundred dollars, and for each subsequent offense a fine of not less than seventy-five nor more than one hundred and fifty dollars.

On complaint being entered the commissioners of pharmacy are hereby empowered to employ an analyst or chemical expert, whose duty it shall be to examine into the so-claimed adulteration, substitution, or alteration and report upon the result of his investigation; and if said report justify such action the commission shall duly cause the prosecution of the offender, as provided in this law.

Sec. 13. No person shall sell at retail any poisons commonly recognized as such, and especially aconite, arsenic, belladonna, biniodide of mercury, carbolic acid, chloral hydrate, chloroform, conium, corrosive sublimate, creosote, croton oil, cyanide of potassium, digitalis, hydrocyanic acid, laudanum, morphine, nux vomica, oil of bitter almonds, opium, oxalic acid, strychnine, sugar of lead, sulphate of zinc, white precipitate, red precipitate, without affixing to the box, bottle, vessel, or package containing the same, and the wrapper or cover thereof, a label bearing the name of the article and the word "poison" distinctly shown, with the name and place of business of the seller; who shall not deliver any of said poisons to any person under the age of fifteen years, nor shall he deliver any of said poisons to any person without satisfying himself that such poison is to be used for a legitimate purpose: *Provided*, That nothing herein contained shall apply to the dispensing of physicians' prescriptions of any of the poisons or articles aforesaid. It shall be the duty of the person vending any of the poisons aforesaid, before delivering the same to the purchaser, to cause an entry to be made in a book kept for that purpose, stating the date of sale, the name and address of the purchaser, the name and quantity of the poison sold, and the name of the dispenser; and such book shall always be open for inspection by the proper authorities and shall be preserved for reference for at least two years. Any person failing to comply with the requirements of this section shall be liable to a penalty of ten dollars for each and every offense.

Sec. 14. All suits for the recovery of the several penalties prescribed in this act shall be prosecuted in the name of the Territory of Wyoming, in any court having jurisdiction, and it shall be the duty of the prosecuting attorney of the county where such offense is committed to prosecute all persons violating the provisions of this act upon proper complaint being made. All penalties collected under the provisions of this act shall inure to the commissioners of pharmacy.

SEC. 15. All registered pharmacists under this act, while actively engaged in conducting any pharmacy or store for retailing drugs, medicines, or poisons, shall be exempt from serving on any jury.

SEC. 16. Chapter two of title thirty-four of the revised statutes of Wyoming is hereby repealed.

SEC. 17. This act shall take effect and be in force from and after its passage.

www.ingramcontent.com/pod-product-compliance
Lightning Source LLC
Chambersburg PA
CBHW030338170426
43202CB00010B/1164